DISCOVER THE MIRACLES THAT CAN TOUCH US ALL IN

THE HEALING ART OF QI GONG

more

D1263013

THE
HEALING
ART OF
QI GONG

Ancient Wisdom from
a Modern Master

MASTER HONG LIU
WITH PAUL PERRY

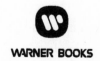

WARNER BOOKS

NEW YORK   BOSTON

The information in this book can be a valuable addition to your doctor's advice but it is not intended to replace the services of trained health professionals. You are advised to consult with your health-care professional with regard to matters relating to your health, and in particular regarding symptoms that may require diagnosis or immediate attention.

This prescription of Chinese herbal formulas is an art form more specific to the individual than are most Westerns prescription medicines. The prescriptions listed in this book were designed only for the individuals described. If you wish to use herbal formulas, it is medically necessary to consult an Oriental doctor and obtain a prescription tailored to your needs.

Master Hong Liu received formal medical training in China but he is not a licensed medical doctor in the United States.

Warner Books is not responsible for the delivery or content of information or materials offered by the author and other sources listed on pages 285–286.

Copyright © 1997 by Dr. Hong Liu, Alice Liu, and Paul Perry
All rights reserved.

Warner Books
Hachette Book Group USA
1271 Avenue of the Americas
New York, NY 10020

Visit our Web site at www.HachetteBookGroupUSA.com.

Printed in the United States of America

First Trade Edition: September 1999
10 9 8 7 6

Warner Books and the "W" logo are trademarks of Time Warner Inc. or an affiliated company. Used under license by Hachette Book Group USA, which is not affiliated with Time Warner Inc.

The Library of Congress has cataloged the hardcover edition as follows:

Liu, Hong.
      Mastering miracles : the healing art of Qi gong as taught by a
master / Dr. Hong Liu, with Paul Perry.
        p. cm.
      ISBN 0-446-52030-6
      1. Ch'i kung 2. Exercise therapy. I. Perry, Paul.
      II. Title.
RA781.8.L58 1996
613.7'1—dc20   96-18309
                                          CIP

ISBN 0-446-67347-1 (pbk.)

Book design and composition by L&G McRee

Acknowledgments

I would like to express my deep thanks:

To my Master, Master Kwan, for all he imparted to me.

To my co-author, Paul Perry, and my wife, Alice Liu, who made this book happen.

To my U.S. apprentices—Jason Chen, Kevin Chen, Kenny Wong, John Yu, Lee Waddell, Wes Graham, Basil Shehady, Lynn Thomas, Jessica Chung, Julie Ko, Bo Barkhordar, Sam Hoony, and Sammy Phan—for their assistance with translation, review, and other tasks.

To Alisa Kao, with the assistance of Grace Kao, for illustrations true to the forms.

To my attorney and apprentice, Arthur Azdair.

To all the others, past and present, who have made this book possible.

Contents

CONTENTS

Qi [*chee*]: The fundamental life force that permeates all things. Qi connects and animates everything in the universe. When the flow of Qi is impaired, we have disease. When it flows easily, we have perfect health.

Qi Gong: The art and science of using breath, movement, mind, and meditation to cleanse, strengthen, and circulate the blood and vital life energy.

Foreword

It is important to note that I was sitting down when I first met Dr. Hong Liu, master of Qi Gong.

I was at a conference on alternative therapies when word began to spread about this Chinese doctor who could diagnose physical problems just by looking at a person. The testimonies were hard for me to believe:

"You just sit there and he doesn't say a word," said one woman. "He looks at you and then puts marks on the outline of a person that is drawn on paper. Without question he marked areas where I have pain."

"He did the same thing to me," said a Los Angeles businessman. "I couldn't believe it. I brought several friends to see Dr. Liu and he did the same thing with them."

"I watched him do it with about a dozen people," said Dannion Brinkley, whose story I wrote about in *Saved by the Light*, a *New York Times* bestseller for almost a year. "One after another he diagnosed people he had never seen before. You have to try it. This is the future of alternative medicine."

Why not? There was literally no time like the present for me. Four months earlier I had torn a ligament in my left knee. Now I had a painful right ankle that was tight and swollen because I had been overcompensating for my knee injury. In addition my neck was sore from writing in an awkward position on the computer. On top of that, deadlines, stress, and too much coffee had left me with a stomachache. All of these were pretty typical American complaints. None of them, I might add, was obvious to the naked eye.

Just for fun, I decided to go see Dr. Liu.

The room in which he was seeing patients was empty. I sat down and waited. Soon Dr. Liu breezed in and sat down in front of me. He said a few words of greeting in Chinese and never asked what was wrong with me. In a moment he was scanning my body and making notes on a generic outline of a man that was held in his clipboard. He put an X over my left knee, one by my right ankle, another on my neck, and a big one across my stomach.

When he finished, one of his students sat next to him to interpret the results.

"Your knee is very bad and may require structural surgery," he said, almost apologetically. "Your ankle is no big deal. You are stepping on it wrong and you just need to make it limber. Your neck, too. Get some massage and move your head more during the day or you will get headaches."

Dr. Liu called to one of his students in Chinese and soon a steaming cup of green tea was brought to him. He held his hand above the cup and concentrated on it. Then he handed it to me and spoke to his assistant.

"He says he has charged it with Qi," he told me. "You are to drink it as fast as possible and concentrate on how it feels and where the heat goes. That'll help cure your stomachache.

Oh, yes, take it easy, too. Stress will then go away. That always helps stomach problems."

And so it did.

If there is one concept that comes up in all forms of Chinese medicine it is that of Qi, or vital energy. Qi is the very backbone of the Chinese healing arts. It refers to the energy of the universe that is channeled from nature and runs through all of us. To have Qi is to be alive, while to have none is to be dead.

Although Western physicians consider Qi an abstraction, for the Chinese it is a reality on which many treatments are based. Acupuncturists, for instance, refer to hundreds of points on the human body where they can insert needles and manipulate Qi to treat illness. The effectiveness of that ancient healing art was brought home to the American public in the 1970s, when, on a trip to China, newspaper columnist Stewart Alsop had an emergency appendectomy using only acupuncture as an anesthetic. After he wrote a column about the experience, interest in acupuncture surged and has been on the rise ever since.

Qi Gong also relies on the manipulation of this vital energy. This is done through "meridians," channels that pass through all the vital organs of the body. There are twelve of these meridians, which correspond to twelve organs. These meridians are interconnected, so that one runs into the other and passes through the body like an invisible river of energy. Anyone can learn simple exercises to manipulate his or her own Qi. This practice is known as *internal* Qi Gong.

Qi Gong masters can see this energy. They can tell when a person has too much Qi or too little, and they can use this information to diagnose illness. They can also project their own Qi externally to change the flow of energy through a patient's meridians.

Although this "external Qi Gong" sounds bizarre to the Western ear, even skeptical Harvard physicians who have experienced it personally say they can feel electrical sensations in their bodies when a Qi Gong master projects his healing power onto them. A senior scientist at the National Electro Acoustics Laboratory in Beijing discovered that low-frequency acoustical waves emitted from the hands of Qi Gong masters are one hundred times as powerful as those of the average individual and one thousand times more powerful than those of the elderly or ill.

Scientific research has proven the benefit of these external power projections. In one study conducted in China, three test tubes containing a common bacteria were given to a Qi Gong master. In the one where no Qi projection was done, the population of the bacteria remained the same. In the one where lethal Qi was projected, the number of bacteria dropped by almost fifty percent. In the test tube that received the health-promoting dose of Qi, the number of bacteria increased by more than thirty percent.

Dr. Liu has accomplished the same thing with cancer cells. In a laboratory at Shanghai Red Cross Hospital he emitted lethal Qi to kill cancer cells that were being cultured in a petri dish. In the dish that received the projected Qi, most of the cancer cells died. The cancer cells in a control dish that received no Qi flourished. Dr. Liu jokingly refers to this as "radiation, Qi Gong style."

The National Institutes of Health is interested enough in the many treatments of Qi Gong that it has begun several studies under the auspices of the Office of Alternative Medicine. Other countries and some institutions in the Western world already have a head start on the NIH. A large database of research covering both external and internal Qi Gong already exists. Hundreds of studies show its positive effects on illness:

- At the National Yang Ming Medical College in Taipei, Qi Gong masters emitted two different types of Qi energy into cultures of human cells to see how Qi affects biochemistry. The cells that received "peaceful mind" Qi had substantially higher growth rates, DNA synthesis, and respiration rates than cells that did not receive Qi. The cells that received "destroying mind" Qi, meanwhile, had greatly decreased growth rates, slower DNA synthesis, and lower respiration rates.

- Immunity can be improved through Qi Gong treatments. At the Shanghai Academy of Traditional Chinese Medicine, blood samples from humans were treated in three different ways: Qi from a Qi Gong master was emitted into eight samples for thirty minutes. Nonpractitioners of Qi Gong imitated the actions of Qi Gong masters into a second batch of blood samples. Finally, a control group of blood samples were untreated.

   The Qi emitted by the Qi Gong masters increased the proliferation of T-cells (immune system cells that are attacked by the HIV virus) by thirty percent over the control group. It also increased the production of interleukin-2 (another substance vital to immunity) by fifty-one percent and the function of natural killer cells (cells that destroy virus-infected cells) by twenty percent.

- External Qi has been shown to kill cancerous tissue and shrink tumors implanted in rats. In one study conducted at the Jiangsu Provincial Research Institute of Traditional Chinese Medicine, a Qi Gong master emitted Qi into ten rats with tumors for twenty to thirty minutes per day while a control group of ten rats went untreated. The tumors in the treated rats shrank by almost fifty percent, while the tumors in the untreated rats remained the same. The peripheral lymph nodes of the treated rats became larger, and their hemoglobin count was much higher—signs that their bodies were fighting the cancer.

These are just a few of the hundreds of scientific studies that have been conducted on the effects of Qi on human and animal biochemistry. We will discuss many more of these in this book.

It is important to note, however, that Qi Gong and the other forms of traditional Chinese medicine covered in this book have been developed and tested over three thousand years. That means that these medical treatments have been used on tens of millions of people and have withstood the test of time. Treatments that don't work don't last more than a few years, let alone thousands of years.

There is nothing paranormal about administering external Qi, according to Dr. Liu. Almost anyone who wants to devote twenty years to the study of Qi Gong, as he has, can master it. Internal Qi Gong, however, is a different matter. This is treatment of disease that one does for oneself. It consists of specific exercises, herbal remedies, and foods that function as medicine. People get information about Qi Gong from masters like Dr. Hong Liu, but they carry out the treatment themselves and are ultimately responsible for their own medical destiny.

The practitioners of Chinese medicine believe that most illnesses are self-inflicted. If this can be interpreted to mean that disease is caused by lifestyle, then the Chinese are correct. Studies conducted by the National Institutes of Health have confirmed that six out of ten illnesses in America could be avoided, and even remedied, through such lifestyle changes as eating less, exercising more, cutting back on alcohol consumption, reducing stress, and eliminating tobacco.

Qi Gong masters and other practitioners of traditional

Chinese medicine know that the surest way to alter the course of a disease is to give the patients herbal remedies, a strong dose of external Qi, and the tools to fight his or her own battle against disease. This philosophy has been stated by many doctors and philosophers of Asia, including the poet Lao-tzu, who wrote: "My life is in my hands, not in the control of heaven and earth."

In essence, Qi Gong combines all the elements of medicine and psychology and includes active involvement by the patient to mobilize all the aspects of healing. As Dr. David Eisenberg of Harvard University wrote in *Encounters with Qi* (W. W. Norton, 1985): "Qi Gong combines aerobic, isometric, and isotonic exercise with the relaxation response, meditation, guided imagery, and probably several unrecognized behavioral techniques. It evokes simultaneously almost every behavioral intervention known to Western medicine. Perhaps the synergistic effect of these techniques can alter human physiology, especially the body's immune system, and thus influence the natural course of illness."

The Healing Art of Qi Gong explores the basics of Qi Gong to create a guide for greater health, the Chinese way.

And there is no better person in the United States to provide this information than Dr. Hong Liu. After graduating from medical school, Dr. Liu became intrigued by Master Kwan, a Qi Gong master who treated the illnesses of China's highest government officials.

After years of studying under Master Kwan, Dr. Liu became one of China's top cancer specialists, treating thousands of patients successfully with a combination of Eastern and Western medicine. He became the Qi Gong master for the Chinese National Assembly and treated the highest members of the Communist Party. He came to the United States in 1990 when a grateful patient left him a large amount of southern California property in her will. He renounced any claim to the property, but after spending a few weeks in California, Dr. Liu realized that he could not return to his hometown of Shanghai. "Without a doubt, America needed Qi Gong," he says. "Being here made me feel like a missionary in a pagan land."

I have spent considerable time with Dr. Liu as he tirelessly performs his alternative healing mission. Unlike most doctors' offices, his is wide open. A large exercise and waiting room is divided from the consultation area by a cherrywood credenza. On top of this richly lacquered piece of furniture is an ornate jar filled with a pungent herbal remedy called "cup of a thousand sips."

Pictures occupy the rest of the table, including a framed photograph of Goldie Hawn gratefully hugging Dr. Liu.

Beyond the room divider is a cherrywood table surrounded by sturdy and comfortable chairs with deep cushions and wide arms. It is in such a chair at the head of the table that Dr. Liu sits when he performs his diagnoses.

This environment creates an air of openness among Dr. Liu's patients. Young people and old talk freely about the reasons they came to see "the master." It is not uncommon to hear stories about cures that seem simply miraculous.

One day, for instance, I met a lovely young woman with curly red hair and the robust ruddy skin of the Irish. I introduced myself and asked her why she was there.

"I have ovarian cancer," she stated matter-of-factly.

I found her story to be typical of Dr. Liu's patients. This patient, whom I will call Marie, had been diagnosed two years earlier with this deadly disease. Doctors found a large tumor on her ovaries and prescribed chemotherapy.

Marie was depressed by the diagnosis. She became lethargic and began to gain weight. Soon she was on a diet of junk food and was thirty pounds overweight. After a while she quit her job and found herself doing nothing but watching television and eating.

"It was as though I was just waiting," she said.

Marie heard about Dr. Liu and decided to try one of his Qi Gong classes. Her tumor had been eight centimeters for a year now. Nothing, it appeared, would help it shrink.

"I got into Qi Gong for exercise," she said. "I began by doing exercises with a class and then I advanced to free-form Qi Gong."

Marie liked the Qi Gong exercises. They helped her relax and gave her a sense of control over herself. Less skeptical now, Marie decided to let Dr. Liu treat her.

He has her do a number of things. Daily she does one to three hours of Qi Gong exercises. "I do them quietly or with soft music," she said. "And I usually do them before bed to help me sleep."

Her herbal regimen was quite extensive: In addition to two different herbal teas, she was taking capsules made of crab shells twice a day and drinking a mushroom soup daily.

In the several months that Dr. Liu has treated her, Marie has lost thirty pounds through dietary changes and exercise. She has also gained back much of the muscle tone that she had lost. Most important, though, is this: Her tumor has shrunk to half the size it was before Dr. Liu began treatments. Now her oncologist has postponed her chemotherapy indefinitely, seeing no reason to treat a shrinking tumor.

"I keep feeling better and of course the results are good," said Marie. "Frankly, I would be happy to live like this for another forty years. But if my cancer goes away, this will be no spontaneous remission. I have worked hard at it."

Another patient who "works at it" is a woman I'll call Debbie, a spirited mother who was afflicted by a rare disease called thrombocytosis. For some unknown reason, Debbie's body was producing far too many platelets, a substance that gives the blood its ability to clot.

For several months she had been feeling lethargic and had symptoms of slurred speech, poor vision, and inability to concentrate. Her family doctor was unable to diagnose the problem and wrote it off to the stress of motherhood. Oddly enough, it was a psychic healer who eventually diagnosed Debbie's disease. On the advice of a friend, Debbie visited the woman in Fontana, California, who told her that "little round things" were circulating in her blood and getting stuck in the vessels.

Debbie went back to her doctor and insisted on a more serious blood analysis. When the results came back, she was immediately referred to a hematologist at UCLA who provided a name for the illness the psychic had described. That doctor prescribed a drug called Hydrea to reduce her platelet count. This is a drug used to treat leukemia and other forms of cancer, and its role is to reduce the production of platelets by the spleen. It had no effect on Debbie's platelet count, which was now as high as one million—some four times higher than normal.

Once again she sought alternative healing, this time from Dr. Liu. She had heard about him from a friend and thought that maybe he could help her. Dr. Liu did not know her Western diagnosis, yet in his initial diagnosis he could tell that Debbie had a swollen spleen and liver. He prescribed a course of therapy that would unblock the liver meridian and reduce the swelling in those vital organs. This included the administration of external Qi, potent herbal teas, and special exercises aimed at reducing the swelling of the liver and spleen, and unblocking the meridian that nourishes the organs. He would not let her stop taking the Hydrea, saying that her body would respond better with a dual approach.

After her treatments from Dr. Liu, her platelet count began to drop. She is now back to normal and continues her Qi Gong treatments to stay that way.

When her doctor at UCLA saw what was happening, he postulated about what had occurred. There is some speculation in the medical community, he said, that this particular blood disorder is caused by a faulty brain signal. Maybe Dr. Liu's Qi Gong treatments had somehow corrected that faulty signal and brought the blood back into balance.

Whatever she was doing, she should keep doing it, her doctor told her.

Like Debbie's physician, I find myself speculating upon the mechanism by which Qi Gong works. Having been raised under the Western model of medicine, I am more and more curious about Qi Gong, especially when it appears to work with great efficacy.

- What is the healing energy that passes from a Qi Gong master to his patient?
- Can specialized exercises really direct a healing force to an area of the body that needs it?
- We already know that the mind is the healer of many diseases. Do we all have a medicine chest on our shoulders that exceeds our expectations?
- Are there truly energy fields flowing through and surrounding our bodies that can affect our health by their very flow? Are they, as the Chinese believe, really as important as the circulation of blood when it comes to good health?

These are all questions that are answered in this book, which is divided into two parts. The first part, "Becoming a Master," shows the path that led Dr. Liu to the mysterious and sometimes mystical world of the Qi Gong masters. The second part of the book, "Studies in Healing," examines the healing methods of these ancient medical arts by showing Dr. Liu's approach to a number of different diseases. Included in that section are Qi Gong exercises, herbal remedies, and "healing recipes," meals that have long been used in China to heal illness.

This book is written in the first person from Dr. Liu's point of view. I did this as a service to the reader, who in my opinion should experience the full force of a person like Dr. Liu. It is my hope that as you read this book it will be as though you are sitting in a room with this amazing man as he tells you his story himself, with no one else to stand in the way.

I still have many questions about Qi Gong, but that is the way it is supposed to be. Scientific inquiry is a wellspring of questions, with answers and questions following one into another, in an endless process. With that realization, it can be comforting to remember the words of the Taoist philosopher who wrote: "The way to long life and health is quite simple and often escapes the attention of those who look for complicated solutions."

—PAUL PERRY

PART I

Becoming a Master

1

The Master

It was my good fortune to be raised in the presence of healers.

My mother was the director of medical care and hospitals in Shanghai, an enormous job that could only be accomplished by someone with boundless energy and deep curiosity about medical treatments of all kinds. She spoke about the causes and cures of illness almost all the time, no matter who was around. One of my first memories is of my mother talking about the importance of public health to the strength of the nation.

When it came to health, she was very open-minded. "A good doctor has to trust his intuition because some things can be sensed but not explained," she told me. "It is important to rely on science, but even more important to remember that intuition usually comes first and then leads to science."

It was a rare day when our house was not teeming with doctors of all kinds. They would stop by after their day's work and drink some tea in the living room of our French colonial–style home in downtown Shanghai. Sometimes the room would fill up and the conversation would become very lively, as doctors talked about difficult cases or some of the many public health hazards that plagued China in the early years of the People's Republic.

As a young man I benefited from these debates. I realized that there were many paths to healing, not just one. A particular path might work for most people but not everyone. Sometimes new treatments would be discovered, or rediscovered, and people who were thought to be hopeless would now become treatable.

A good doctor was aware of all the paths and open to trying new ones, especially if a patient was otherwise on a road to nowhere. Sometimes patients take several different paths to find healing. Sometimes they never find it, no matter how many paths they take. The role of a good doctor is to know all the alternatives and help the patients understand where they are going in their search for health.

Raised in this kind of environment, there was never any question that I would become a medical doctor. I enrolled in the Military Medical College, where my studies were focused on allopathic medicine, the type of medicine familiar to most Americans, also known as Western medicine. But in addition, we were trained in Chinese herbal medicine, which is the use of nature's pharmacopoeia in healing diseases.

During medical school and into my practice, I returned home to immerse myself in the ongoing debate about health and healing. This debate had now expanded to include healers who were beyond the scope of "usual" medicine. During the Cultural Revolution, Chairman Mao's wife had ordered that all ancient medical traditions be banned so that he could gain tighter control over Chinese society. But my mother had bravely spoken out in favor of traditional medicine, an act that convinced the responsible officials to exempt them from extinction.

Many Qi Gong masters, as well as other healers, had been released from prison because of my mother's intervention and they immediately recognized her as a friend. Now they, too, came to drink tea and mingle with the medical doctors.

The Chinese say that "where Qi Gong masters gather, so do patients." This was certainly true at our house, where a crowd of sick people arrived with each visiting master.

There was one Qi Gong master, however, who outdrew all the others. Every time he came from his home in the mountains of southern China, the house filled with people who wanted to be examined by him. Sometimes the house became so full that it was almost impossible for me to get across the living room and into my own bedroom. I would stand and watch as he diagnosed and treated dozens of people.

The examinations he conducted were amazing. He never asked what ailment the patient had. Instead he looked at the person briefly as though they were some kind of curious flower. Then he would just blurt out the patient's illness and where it bothered the patient most. He told patients their symptoms and could even tell what problems they had had in the past and whether their illness was hereditary.

After giving them external Qi treatments, using his own energy to unblock theirs, he would show people techniques and exercises they could do to manipulate their own Qi. Sometimes he would write a prescription for herbs.

When he was finished, he moved on to the next patient, and so on until he was finished with everyone.

One night he was pressed for time and did something that was new to me. He asked a group of about twenty patients to sit down and concentrate on their illness. Then he began to meditate, projecting his Qi on the group for about fifteen minutes. Suddenly some of the people began to laugh while others began to cry. They spoke of sensations that were like electrical charges inside their bodies. Others said they could feel things move inside of them. Almost everyone came away filled with vitality, as though each person had been recharged with life.

I was in awe of what I saw. It was as though he were pulling energy from the universe and transmitting it to those who needed it. One night after he left I told my mother that I was stunned by what I saw this man do.

"We are constantly using science to search for the meaning of life and the power of the universe," I said to my mother. "Yet this man seems to possess the power of life without science."

What she said confused me at the time, although I came to understand it perfectly later.

"What this master possesses isn't magic," she said. "It is just science that has not yet been examined."

I began to find out more about this Master Kwan, although much about him remains a mystery to me, even to this day. I was told that he lived outside of Canton high on a mountain in a cave. Even though the path to his home was steep and somewhat difficult, the citizens of Canton and surrounding areas flocked to see him. It was common for him to start seeing patients early in the morning and to be working with them until well after sundown.

The only people who did not trek up the mountain were high government officials. Instead they sent messengers to make the trip for them. When they requested his presence, Master Kwan reluctantly ventured off the mountain. Even a master does not say no to the government of China.

When he was treating government officials in Shanghai he usually stayed at my mother's house. Then, at any time of day or night, we could expect a black government car to appear in the alley and take Master Kwan away. Usually he would be taken to the offices or private residences of the officials to conduct treatments. On rare occasions, however, government officials came to our house for treatment. One such occasion came when the mayor of Shanghai came for treatment of a problem that he refused to talk about in advance. His assistant was mysterious when asked why the mayor was coming. At first he would say nothing about the mayor's medical condition. Then, when my mother pressed him, the nervous young man would say only that the mayor had dealt with a number of Western-trained physicians, but to no avail.

"It is you who must ask him what the problem is," said the assistant. "It is too personal for me to tell you."

Word of his visit got around, and on the day of the appointment, the house began to fill with people. Not only did medical doctors show up, but also our neighbors and patients of Master Kwan. By the time the mayor arrived, there was a large group of spectators filling the living room.

At the appointed hour, three official cars arrived in back of the house. Without knocking, four bodyguards walked through the door and began searching the residence. When they saw that the living room was full of spectators, they demanded that everyone clear out. Master Kwan refused.

"You don't dare tell my people to leave," he said. "These are my invited guests."

The bodyguards began to argue, but Master Kwan dug in his heels. The master had a mind of his own, a trait not common among the Chinese people in those days. As he argued with the government bodyguards, everyone in the room became very quiet and nervous. Still Master Kwan persevered.

"If these people cannot stay, then your boss cannot come in and be treated," shouted Master Kwan. He had been jailed during the Cultural Revolution and had a sincere dislike of the police, even those in the glorified form of bodyguards. He opposed their authority whenever he could.

"Why don't you leave?" he shouted. "Then there would be more room than we would know what to do with."

Before the bodyguards could respond to this insult, the mayor walked into the room. He was an enormous man who practically filled the doorway when he appeared. It was rare in China to see someone who was so heavy, and everyone gaped openly at his girth.

At first he was surprised to see so many people. Then he began to smile. He told my mother that he was honored that so many of his people were interested in his well-being. He shook a few hands and waved to people in the back of the room and remarked about how cold it had been that winter in Shanghai.

Master Kwan had him sit down and they began to chat. Although I counted more than fifty people in the room, not a sound was uttered as the two talked.

What happened over the course of their conversation was amazing.

Almost as soon as the mayor sat down, he began to perspire. I noticed beads of sweat forming on his forehead and soon he took a handkerchief out of his pocket and was wiping it over his face. How strange, I thought. My own forehead felt cool and it was even so cold in the room that you could see the breath of some of the people near the front door.

I turned my attention to the mayor. He was perspiring more profusely now and was even unbuttoning his shirt. As I listened to the conversation I realized that they had not even begun to address the medical condition, whatever it was, that had brought the mayor in the first place.

The treatment was supposed to take only thirty minutes. When that time had passed, however, the mayor excused himself to go to the bathroom and then returned and continued talking to Master Kwan. After forty minutes he stood up and removed his jacket, which caused a buzz in the room since it was so cold already. A few minutes later he removed his shirt, which was now damp with perspiration. Very strange, I thought. The mayor of Shanghai is sitting in a cold room with only his undershirt on and still he is perspiring!

An hour had passed and the mayor's assistants were beginning to fidget. They had scheduled only thirty minutes for the meeting and were now wondering when he would be finished. One of the assistants stepped forward and whispered to the mayor, who waved him away. "Cancel that meeting," he said. "This is too interesting."

The assistant scurried out of the room to make a telephone call and the mayor went to the bathroom for the second time.

He returned and discussion began about the theories behind Qi Gong. Master Kwan had the mayor's undivided attention. The big man sat on the chair and listened attentively to the master as he talked about the origin and uses of his healing art. As the mayor listened he was perspiring so much that my mother finally gave him a towel.

He went to the bathroom for a third time and returned. An hour and thirty minutes had passed and still no mention had been made of why the mayor had come to see Master Kwan.

The conversation continued and so did the perspiration. I did not know how the mayor could ignore such drenching perspiration, and concluded that he was so impressed with Master Kwan that he did not notice it. He looked like a man who had run a footrace.

After two hours, he went to the bathroom a fourth time. When he returned, Master Kwan stood up and bowed.

"That is the end of your treatment," he said.

"It can't be!" insisted the mayor. "I haven't told you why I came to see you!"

"I know already," insisted Master Kwan. "You came because you are so heavy. You want to lose some weight."

"That's true!" said the mayor. "How did you know?"

Everyone in the room laughed when he said this. The only ones who did not know about Master Kwan's powers of remote diagnosis were the mayor and his entourage.

"Look at what happened here," Master Kwan said, addressing the mayor. "You have been perspiring for two hours. You have gone to the bathroom four times. This will continue all day."

The mayor became very excited. He wanted to sit down and talk more, but his assistants were now demanding that he leave.

"We will talk again soon," said Master Kwan, handing the mayor his shirt.

When the big man left, Master Kwan explained that he had increased the mayor's metabolism. By speeding up all of his bodily processes, Master Kwan made sure the mayor would burn more calories and would lose weight. Doing this had caused the mayor to have diarrhea, which is why he had gone to the bathroom so many times. "That will continue for a couple of days until his body adjusts to the faster metabolism," said Master Kwan.

I could contain myself no longer. "But what did you do to change his metabolism?" I asked. "You never touched him. What did you do to make him sweat?"

Master Kwan nodded like a professor forming his thoughts.

"There are three ways to convey energy," he said. "The most direct way is through acupuncture needles. The second is by touching people in meridian spots. The third and most powerful is by using remote Qi to send the energy directly through the air. That is what I did with the mayor. As we talked, I just pointed my fingers at him and continued with the conversation. The Qi that I emitted raised his metabolism, as you could all see."

He then sat down and demonstrated the position his hands had been in when the mayor was there. His hand was resting on his thigh with his fingers together and pointed at the chair where the mayor had sat.

The next day the mayor called Master Kwan from a train. He was still perspiring and had gone to the bathroom several times that night as the master had said he would. Before he hung up he made another appointment to see the master.

Master Kwan usually said nothing about his visits to high government officials. As with all patients, their cases were considered confidential. It was not uncommon for us to be talking about some government official around the house when the master would say, "I treated him just last week," or "I have visited him and his family many times."

That would usually be the extent of Master Kwan's comments. He knew the power of the government and was very careful to keep information to himself about the people he treated. He had spent a few years in prison for practicing Qi Gong during the Cultural Revolution and would probably have been there still if my mother had not intervened.

He broke this rule of silence only once, and that was to tell about the time he treated the man who had imprisoned him.

He told me this story one night as we drank tea in the living room of our house in Shanghai. We were sitting quietly when he began to chuckle to himself. I ignored it at first, thinking that he was laughing at a private joke. When he laughed a few more times, however, I broke down and intruded.

"What is so funny?" I asked.

"I am just remembering the time I treated the man who put me in jail," he said.

The man was the governor of Guangdong, a very large province in the south of China. He had been among the officials who carried out the orders that all of the traditional physicians be rounded up and imprisoned. Chairman Mao's wife felt that any form of tradition detracted from her husband's communistic goals and ordered that all such practitioners be sent to "reeducation" camps. Master Kwan had spent two years in such a camp. Now the man who had ordered his imprisonment just a few years ago was asking that the master provide for his health.

Master Kwan was very pleasant as he was ushered into the governor's office. He concealed his dislike of this man behind a warm smile and friendly greeting. After looking at him for a moment to do a remote diagnosis, Master Kwan told the governor that he had a blockage in his kidney meridian.

"Because this problem is in your back, I need you to take off your shirt," he said.

The governor did so willingly.

Master Kwan looked at the governor more closely.

"Now you need to take off your pants."

The governor did this as well.

Master Kwan had the governor move out from behind his desk and sit in a chair that was in the middle of the room. Then Master Kwan sat in a chair across from him and removed his shoes.

"Lean back," said Master Kwan. When he did as he was told, the master raised one foot and held it against the nose of the governor. Then he rubbed the toes in a circular motion until the governor shuddered.

Of course this was no treatment. Master Kwan told me that it was his way of teaching the governor humiliation, the sort the master had suffered at the hands of government officials like this governor. But the governor did not know this. He was humiliated by the foot in his face, but had to accept it. After all, was this not the Qi Gong master's way of giving him Qi?

When the "treatment" was over, Master Kwan told the governor that he could put his clothing back on.

"How many more times do you have to do that until I am well?" the governor asked.

Master Kwan thought a moment. "At least five times," he replied. "We must do the exact same thing five more times."

But the extent of the necessary treatment presented a problem, said Master Kwan. For his visit to the governor, Master Kwan had been registered into an ordinary hotel, thinking that treatment would take only one day. For an extended visit, he would require much nicer accommodations, preferably like those found in foreign hotels. "If I don't stay in comfortable quarters"—Master Kwan shrugged— "my Qi weakens."

When he told this to the governor, the politician called his assistant on the telephone. A few telephone calls later, and Master Kwan was registered in the presidential suite of the best hotel in Canton, the capital of Guangdong.

"We have you checked in for five days," the assistant told him.

"There must be some mistake," said Master Kwan, addressing the assistant and the governor. "I did say five treatments. But the treatments are once a week."

For more than a month, Master Kwan lived like a king in the presidential suite. Once a week he was picked up by a driver in a government car and taken to the governor's office, where he unceremoniously pressed his foot into the face of the man who had once put him in jail.

The most ironic thing was this: After five weeks of such treatment, the governor was healed. He felt so much better that he sang the praises of the master to other provincial governors. Now, said Master Kwan, he was being invited to care for other governors.

He had only one requirement: To stick his foot in their faces, the governors had to arrange for him to stay five weeks at the presidential suite of a local hotel.

"Revenge has been very kind to me," he said with a laugh.

One time Master Kwan showed up at our house and was very excited. He had been asked to come down from the mountain by the Chinese Sports Federation. Some international table tennis competitions were just a few weeks away and one of the top competitors had a recurrence of a shoulder and back injury that would prevent him from competing.

This would be a disaster for the Chinese. This athlete was the one great hope for a medal at these games. If he was not able to at least compete, the Chinese would lose face in the international athletic community.

The Sports Federation was now in a panic. When the athlete's pain first began, they thought it would just go away if he took it easy. As it worsened, however, they became increasingly nervous. They sent him to Western-trained medical doctors in Beijing who gave him injections of cortisone and painkillers so he would not miss too much practice. Now the pain was so bad that painkillers did not help. The doctors became nervous and began asking their colleagues about alternative solutions. That was when Master Kwan was suggested.

It was a great honor to be asked to treat an athlete, and Master Kwan knew it. The Sports Federation was so respectful of the master that its officials had agreed to bring this athlete to Shanghai if the master would come up from his mountain home near Canton. Master Kwan was very excited when he showed up at our house. He laughed and talked about the sports injuries he had treated, as he waited for the athletes to arrive. This athlete's problem was typical of table tennis players, who make so many repetitive moves that they strain their joints and spine. Master Kwan had healed such problems before. However, to cure such a well-known athlete would indeed be an honor.

When the player and his trainers arrived, however, Master Kwan did not act honored at all. As the group came into the living room, he turned his back on them and began to talk to his apprentices as though the sports people had not come into the room. Then he talked and joked with me and my brother as the sports entourage stood awkwardly behind him, waiting to be noticed.

Finally he spoke to them. "This athlete has been hurt for some time," he said. "You should have taken his pain more seriously when it first started."

"We did everything we could do," said one of the trainers. He described a litany of treatments that the athlete had gone through, including physical therapy and cortisone injections.

"You missed one," said Master Kwan, turning to face the entourage. "You did not bring him to me."

Standing up, Master Kwan raised his arms slowly over his head like a graceful diver and addressed the athlete. "Do what I am doing," he instructed. The boy raised his arms slowly from his side but got no higher than three-quarters of the way before he grimaced and lowered them again.

"What can you do? What can you do?" pleaded one of the trainers.

"Calm down," demanded Master Kwan. "I tell you he will be fine."

He turned the boy around and touched several spots on his back and shoulders. He did not press hard, but merely put his fingers on particular spots and held them there. As he did this, the tension left the player's face and he appeared to be comfortably asleep.

When the master finished, he stepped back and asked the athlete to raise his hands. This time he raised them over his head. When he experienced no pain, the table tennis player began moving his shoulder through a range of motion that obviously would have been impossible when he first came in the door. Now he was laughing and pretending to play table tennis. He was jumping around the room and swinging his arms like a player at the table.

"No pain?" asked Master Kwan. "Do you feel pain anywhere?"

"None at all," the athlete said, continuing to roll his head and twist his neck.

What I saw shocked me. By this time I had already gone through much of my medical training and I knew that the doctors in charge of the athlete's treatment had done everything by the book, yet it had only served to make things worse. What I was seeing was hard to accept.

Master Kwan left the room and soon returned with a hot herbal patch. He taped this patch on the player's lower back and pressed it against his skin.

"Take that off tomorrow when you get back to Beijing," he told him. "Then just continue to train."

There were literally tears in the trainers' eyes as they saw what had happened. A few weeks later the athlete won the competitions.

That night I could barely sleep. In fact, I did not want to sleep. What I had seen was too exciting to ignore. World-class athletes are treated by the best doctors in the country. We call them the "specialists' specialists" because their knowledge about the human body is so extensive. Yet all of their good work cannot heal this table tennis player's pain. Then in comes a man who claims to draw energy from the universe. He touches the player's neck and back in a few places and the athlete is suddenly healed. How could this be? I wondered. How could I ignore this man and his methods of healing?

The desire to control disease was the reason I was becoming a doctor of medicine. Could this energy medicine be combined with my Western medical knowledge to create a superior form of treatment? Was it, as it appeared to be, a combination of isometric and isotonic exercises, combined with meditation and guided imagery as well as a number of other interventions and techniques that were not yet even recognized by medicine? Was it truly a unifying principle of medicine that had been downplayed in favor of a more mechanical interpretation of the human body?

As I started to doze I was left wondering if seeing this night's demonstration was a blessing or a curse. Should I follow my own intuition and learn more about Qi Gong? Or should I keep my focus on the proven, scientific, Western method of medicine I already understood? I was confused.

I fell asleep for a few hours that night but awoke well before sunrise. My mind was full of the mysteries I had seen that night. I thought more about Qi Gong and how it might relate to my life. I was in the army at this time, which exercised control over everything from my training to my living arrangements. Maybe it was futile to even think that I could study under Master Kwan.

Unable to sleep, I got out of bed and quietly began to pace around the house. We had a hallway with big windows that looked out onto a courtyard. On this particular night the windows were open, and even though it was chilly I could feel puffs of warm air, which puzzled me.

As I reached out to close the window, I saw the source of

the warm wind. There in the garden was Master Kwan. He was practicing martial arts, twirling his arms in graceful sweeps that made him look like frothing waves pounding the shore. With every movement of his arm I could hear a crack as though lightning had struck. There was some kind of force that seemed to produce a maverick wind. I don't know how else to explain it. As he performed his graceful routine, winds blew and swayed the plants and trees around him.

It was impressive, exhilarating, and frightening all at the same time.

I must have been leaning very far out the window, because I gasped and almost fell out when a hand touched my back. It was my mother.

"Do not disturb the master when he is practicing," she said.

She reached past me and pulled the window shut. Still I stood there for a long time.

There was no longer any question in my mind. I had to learn Qi Gong from Master Kwan.

2

The Pinnacle of Qi

There were problems created by my desire to study under Master Kwan. I was an army officer practicing in a military hospital and my life was very rigid. Like the other doctors in my unit, I was expected to be in the hospital at certain times and to perform routine duties. My days consisted of long hours of patient care with very little time to involve myself in anything but the practice of Western medicine.

Medical doctors who did not conform and work diligently within the schedule were reprimanded and sometimes demoted. This was not unreasonable, since there were many sick people and few doctors. Still, I had seen medical miracles performed by Master Kwan and I wanted to study them.

I decided to devote all the time I could to the study of Qi Gong. Because of that decision, Master Kwan was the benefactor of all of my spare time for almost eight years. Believe me when I say that spare time does not come easily to a doctor in China.

Usually I would take vacation time or beg a few sick days so I could catch a train to Canton, about six hundred miles south of Shanghai. This was a long, slow trip aboard a train that was usually crowded and uncomfortable. Because of the demand placed on public transportation in China, people sometimes sit in the aisles and jam the space between the trains. If I got to the train station early enough I would sometimes get a seat. Usually, though, I was late and found myself standing a good portion of the trip.

My voyage to the home of Master Kwan did not end when I arrived in Canton. He lived a number of miles outside the city, high on a mountain called the Golden Cock. It had received that name because it resembled a fighting rooster, one with a sloping back and an alert head with a high, bushy comb.

His home was in a cave at the base of the head. To get there required a long hike up the rooster's back, climbing a path that was well worn from the hundreds of patients who had made this same trip. Sometimes I even passed patients on my way to the master's home. It was not uncommon to see people on crutches struggling up the trail, or to see old people in pain being helped up the mountain by family members. I always felt sympathy for these patients and often wondered why Master Kwan did not meet them at the bottom of the mountain instead of making them take this arduous hike. One time I asked, only to be looked at like I should have known the answer. "The trip to my home is proof that a person truly wants to be healed," he said. "The climb up the mountain is a great motivator."

This was no ordinary cave that Master Kwan occupied. The Qi Gong masters of China have thirty-six sacred mountains in the entire country, each with two sacred caves. These caves have attained their status because they are the source of good Qi from their natural surroundings. Because of the abundance of Qi in these areas, they have been occupied by many grand masters, virtual wizards of Qi Gong.

There are many stories about the powers of these grand masters. Some say they have seen the grand masters move trays of dishes across tables by pointing their fingers and exerting Qi force. Others have seen them illuminate fluorescent lights by holding them in their hands, or crush rocks with their heads. It has been said that their Qi Gong powers extend even after life, and that the flesh of some grand masters does not decay when they die. I have seen proof of this. In one sacred cave that I visited in the Szechwan Province, such a grand master was lying in state. He had been there many years and his flesh had not rotted. There is even one such Qi Gong master in Japan, written about in *Ripley's Believe It or Not*, whose body has not decayed even though he has been dead for many years.

Their powers extend beyond life in other ways, too. The spirits of past masters can be felt and even seen in these sacred caves. Many masters swear that the spirits of past masters return to guide them in their healings.

I have seen one such late master myself. One morning I arose before sunrise to do some of my Qi Gong exercises. I had to leave early that day to catch the train to Shanghai and I wanted to make certain that I performed the exercises before leaving.

As I concentrated on the exercises, I was suddenly aware of being watched. I looked toward the mouth of the cave and noticed a man doing the exercises with me. Since Master Kwan frequently stood in this spot and showed me how to do the exercises properly, I just thought it was him. Later in the morning, however, I found out differently.

"Thank you for getting up so early and instructing me," I said appreciatively when I saw Master Kwan.

"I did not get up," he said. "I was still sleeping."

I told him what happened and how the man mirrored my every move.

"He did the exercises as beautifully as you," I said to Master Kwan.

"Then you are lucky," said the master. "You have seen the spirit of one of this cave's past masters."

Master Kwan's cave was the presidential suite of sacred caves. It was a gift of nature, a place where healing arts were intended to be practiced.

The cave was divided into three sections. The first room in the cave was a large living room where people would come to be treated or to visit. All of the furniture in this room was made from wood and other objects from the mountain. It was decorated with gifts brought by grateful patients and was a virtual museum of art objects from all over the country.

This room alone was worth the climb for many people. A small stream flowed from one of the walls and trickled across the floor into a large pool at the center of the room. Koi and other fish drifted near the pool's surface among many water plants. Foliage surrounded the entire pool and gave a lush setting for the benches where patients drank tea and waited for their treatment after the long climb up the mountain.

Through an archway in the back of this room was the chamber for the apprentices and students. There were usually ten to fifteen underlings in the cave at any given time, which made the living in this room very tight. We had thin mattresses that were placed side by side on the hard dirt floor and were covered with one blanket for warmth. Any personal items we had were kept against the wall so they would not be stepped on in the crowded room.

Even though the living conditions could be described as

grim, Master Kwan considered them necessary. He considered such spartan accommodations an important part of the learning process. "It is difficult to learn Qi Gong, but it is supposed to be," he said. "Valuable knowledge does not come through comfort."

Through an archway in the back of the second chamber was Master Kwan's private quarters. This was an extraordinary room, the likes of which I have never seen since. It was in this room that Master Kwan meditated and slept.

The roof of his quarters glistened with moisture and shone with crystal rocks that reflected their beauty in the amber glow of the candles that Master Kwan used for illumination. Benches and a large table crafted from mountain wood occupied the center of the room. This table was always heaped with medical books. Typical of the books to be found were the medical texts of the Yellow Emperor, a classic medical text called *On the Causes and Symptoms of Diseases* that described hundreds of specific Qi Gong exercises for diseases, and books about the pharmacological effects of various herbs and plants.

Philosophical books also had a place on Master Kwan's table. I remember once reading a line from Lao-tzu that Master Kwan had underlined. It was about the power of breathing and it read like this: "Inhaling and exhaling helps to rid one of the stale and take in the fresh. Moving as a bear and stretching as a bird can result in longevity."

At the back portion of this chamber was the master's bed. As you would expect, this was no ordinary bed. It was a thick layer of straw underneath a thin mattress that was topped with a blanket. The bed was six feet above the floor on a ledge of rock that was reached by steps that nature had cut into the stone.

There was never any question that this cave had been created by nature as a sacred place. To just enter it was to be filled with the energy of the universe. I felt that every time, no matter how tired I was from my long voyage.

For eight years I made voyages to Master Kwan's cave. At least twice a month I scrambled to get out of the hospital early and to the train station. Trains are not so comfortable in China. At certain times of the year, the heat would be so bad that people literally passed out from dehydration. Other times of the year we froze. Groups of strangers huddled together to share body heat. This was a good way to meet people, but not a very pleasant way to travel.

These frequent trips took their physical toll on me. I lost weight and was more susceptible to colds and flu. My first days back from the master's cave were usually spent in a haze of exhaustion. My feet and legs were always tired, too, if not from climbing up and down the mountain, then from standing for long periods at a time during the train trips.

The physical toll these trips took on me was nothing compared to the professional toll. I was always in trouble with my bosses. Even though the doctors who headed my department were understanding and curious about my studies, I was testing the limits of their flexibility. I was always late for work after these trips south and I was always trying to get a few extra days off so I could spend more time with Master Kwan.

There were many reprimands in the early years. I was once even threatened with court-martial for dereliction of my duties as a military medical officer. I remember one time being scolded by a doctor who said that I should be ashamed for studying Qi Gong. "You have just spent five years in medical school. Isn't that enough?"

For me it was not enough. I knew the limits of allopathic medicine and had seen Master Kwan use Qi Gong to go beyond those limits in some cases, and to approach a problem differently in other cases. Since my job was to be a healer, I felt it was my duty to learn this ancient method as best I could.

It was clear that I had taken the difficult path in my life. I could easily have settled into a standard medical practice like the rest of my classmates did. Instead I chose to examine alternative therapies because had seen them work on others.

On top of that, the path to learning Qi Gong was difficult, and one that not everyone could understand. There were always people begging for explanation. One day, for example, I fell asleep during a staff meeting at the hospital. It was just after maybe the tenth time I had made the journey to Master Kwan's cave and I was extremely tired and a little depressed. I was awakened by a colleague who laughed and said that I was spending too much time traveling and not enough time sleeping. Later, however, he talked to me outside the conference room.

"Why are you so interested in Qi Gong?" he asked. "What are you getting out of studying it?"

I told him the truth. "I have not only seen the magic of Qi Gong, but I have also experienced it. I have done a Qi Gong healing myself!"

I told him the story.

On my first trip to see Master Kwan, he showed me some external Qi healing techniques. Specifically, he showed me how to deal with noncancerous lumps and bone breaks, which he felt were particularly responsive to Qi Gong.

I was excited to know these techniques. This was my first trip to the master's cave and already he was showing me methods of healing that I would be able to use in my own practice of medicine.

I came down the mountain after that trip and went quickly to the train station to catch a train back to Shanghai. I put my bag into the overhead luggage rack and sat down heavily in an aisle seat. I had just taken a deep breath and begun to nap when I heard a conductor call out for a doctor. I looked out the window and could see a crowd gathering on the platform. They formed a semicircle around someone who was moaning and holding her leg.

I got up quickly and waved to the conductor. "I am a doctor," I said. He grabbed my arm and pulled me down the aisle and off the train. In a moment I was standing over a young woman who was gripping the top of her foot.

She had come off a step on the platform and twisted her ankle very hard, she said. Her ankle joint was starting to swell and the sound she said had accompanied her twisting fall made me think that a bone at the top of her foot had snapped like a twig.

I knelt down and removed her shoe. She was in agony by now and had tears streaming down her face. The members of her family who had come to meet her looked greatly concerned, and everyone else was looking at me in anticipation of what I would do.

The fact was, I did not know exactly what to do. It seemed obvious to me that there was some kind of bone break that would have to be dealt with by a surgeon. Even if that was not true, however, there was a nasty sprain that was extremely painful and getting worse.

"What are you going to do?" asked the conductor.

Frankly I did not know. Then suddenly I remembered the lesson in healing that Master Kwan had given me only the night before.

"If there is obviously an energy blockage in an area of the body, you can break through it by touching the meridian points that are above and below," he said. "Then charge it with Qi energy. That will improve the circulation of both Qi and blood."

Remembering what the master had said, I pulled the woman's pants leg up and found the meridian points. She was in extreme pain and was still crying. The swelling had continued and was now accompanied by a blue-and-red bruise on her ankle.

I put my fingers on the meridian points on her leg and the bottom of the injured foot. Then I concentrated on increasing the flow of Qi energy into her meridian points.

As I did this, her sobbing stopped. Everyone watched as the swelling in her ankle began to decrease. As I continued to administer Qi through the meridian points, the pain diminished. Soon she was rotating her ankle and wiggling her toes.

I have done it, I thought to myself. I have used Qi Gong to heal. I was very excited, but I tried to act as though I had done this many times. "Does that fell better?" I asked.

"It does!" said the woman.

She was helped to her feet by her father, who continued to hold her hands as she tested her foot. She put a little weight on the foot and then—able to withstand that—put her full weight down. Then she walked around in a circle, smiling at the startled spectators.

"Thank you, Doctor," she said, gripping my hands.

I nodded and walked down the platform toward the train car in which I had been riding. I was stunned and speechless. My first Qi Gong healing left me with a feeling that I have never experienced either before or since. I am sure it is the feeling that a caterpillar has when he grows wings and becomes a butterfly.

"Master, Master," said a voice behind me as I climbed upon the train platform. "My hand is frozen. Can you fix it, too?"

I looked back to see an old man holding up his hand, which was gnarled by arthritis. For a moment I thought about getting off the train and attempting to treat this gentleman. Had I just been lucky? I wondered. Should I dare try to heal two people with Qi Gong?

The train made my decision for me. The whistle blew and a moment later the big wheels began to lurch forward.

"I will be back," I shouted to the old man. "I will do what I can to help you then."

I sat down in my seat and took a deep sigh. I was tired, but I could not sleep. Every time I closed my eyes I saw the swelling in the woman's ankle going down. . . . I saw the startled people who watched my first Qi Gong procedure. . . . I saw the hopeful old man holding up his crippled hand as we left the station.

"I experienced firsthand the power of Qi Gong," I told my colleague as we stood in the hallway of the hospital. "If you saw such healing, wouldn't you try to master it, too?"

The story I told my colleague was the only "magic" that happened to me for some time. After I healed the woman on the train platform, my time with Master Kwan became very different. Maybe he saw a change in me that he did not like. Perhaps I had become too cocky and began acting as though Qi were mine and not something that came to me from the universe. Perhaps Master Kwan thought I was no longer aware of the important and humbling words of Lao-tzu, the contemporary of Confucius, who wrote:

There is a thing confusedly formed,
Born before heaven and earth,
Silent and void,
It stands alone and does not change,
Goes round and does not weary.
It is capable of giving birth to the world.
I know not its name
So I style it "the way" . . .

Man models himself on earth,
Earth on heaven,
Heaven on the way,
And the way on that which is naturally so.

Whatever it was, Master Kwan turned his back on me. In the end, however, this was the best learning experience of my life.

The next time I went to the cave I was filled with pride. I told Master Kwan about the woman on the train platform and about the man who begged me to help him with his hand. Master Kwan looked very hard into my face as I told this story. His gaze was so intense that I began to perspire. I pulled a handkerchief from my pocket and wiped my face as I continued to talk. I could tell, however, that he was not listening and I became very embarrassed. When I finished my story he turned away and began talking to an apprentice.

I knew I had done something wrong, but I did not know what it was.

For the remainder of my stay I was asked to do "cave work," which was simply cleaning up after patients and sweeping the floor.

I thought this would change the next time I went up to the cave. I arrived full of enthusiasm and ready to learn. This time, however, Master Kwan would not even talk to me. Instead I was taken aside by an apprentice, who told me that since I was a student, I must do the work of a student. Then he handed me a broom.

I was angry. The apprentice who had ordered me to sweep the floors was a peasant named Wang. He was studying Qi Gong so he could practice the traditional Chinese medicine in the rural region where he came from. How could Master Kwan have asked this uneducated person to give me such demeaning orders?

I took the broom, but not without glaring angrily at the apprentice. For the next three days I swept the cave floor very hard.

And so it went. After several such trips I was becoming disheartened. These trips were hard on me. For one thing, no one in mainland China makes very much money, and I was no exception. I was spending almost all of my pay on train tickets to study with the master. I was also taxing my reputation. Leaving work early and returning sometimes days late was not an acceptable thing to do in Communist China. Master Kwan knew that I was putting a lot on the line. Did it not matter to him?

I went up to the mountain again, filled with resolve and ready to confront Master Kwan about my fruitless visits to his cave. For a day I did cave work, building up courage as I swept and cleaned. Finally, on the morning of the second day, I confronted Master Kwan with my frustration.

"Why won't you teach me anything?" I demanded.

"Because you are too greedy," said the master. "You haven't learned the true lessons of what I taught you and you are asking for more."

I was puzzled, which must have been obvious in my expression.

"Rule number one," said Master Kwan, holding up his index finger. "Your worst enemy is greed. Why do you want to learn Qi Gong? What is the purpose?"

The question left me speechless. I could only shrug.

"Your purpose is to treat patients," he said. "You have treated only one patient. What about the other patients? Have you used it at the hospital in Shanghai? No. Have you used it with Western medicine? No. You keep coming back wanting to learn more, but you are not using the knowledge that I have already given you. You have treated one patient with Qi Gong. Why should you get more knowledge?"

My face burned with embarrassment as the other students and apprentices chuckled. This was not the lesson I had hoped to receive from the master. I bowed my head in shame and vowed silently to do better.

When I returned to Shanghai I secretly treated ten patients at the hospital with Qi Gong, without them knowing about it. Most of these were patients with chronic illnesses like arthritis or ulcers. The usual medications were being used, but they were not totally effective in relieving pain. When they asked me for help, I used the knowledge I had received from Master Kwan and found it to be effective in reducing the pain these people were experiencing. Even this minor success drove me to want to learn more.

Once again I went to the mountain. I stood before Master Kwan and reported my success. "I have treated thirty patients with Qi Gong," I lied. "I have done what you asked me to do."

I had blown up the story to try to make myself look better in the eyes of Master Kwan. Thirty people sounded better than ten. Surely he would teach me more about Qi Gong now, I thought. I realized what a mistake this had been in the very next moment.

"You are not being too realistic," he said, looking me directly in the eyes. "You tell me about thirty people, but you have only used it with about ten people. I know this."

The students and apprentices laughed. I later realized that they were not laughing at me, but because they, too, had been caught in such "little lies" by the master and found it funny when a new student discovered the master's ability to read their thoughts like words on a page. "You cannot hide truth from a Qi Gong master," Wang said to me later. Still I was humiliated at being caught. I began to stammer as I tried to explain to Master Kwan.

"I am under a lot of pressure," I said. "The other doctors

in my unit do not think that I should be studying Qi Gong. They think it is beneath a doctor to do such things."

"I understand what you are thinking about," said Master Kwan. "You are thinking that you are a medical doctor and you don't want to use traditional Chinese methods of healing. You are thinking about your name. Your medical degree gives you a golden bough, because you can always make a good living. You don't want to risk that more than you already have. This presents a problem, since you have seen with your own eyes the full power of Qi Gong. You know that it can heal illnesses. You know that, combined with Western medicine, the two can sometimes heal better than either one alone. You have seen all of this with your own eyes, so you know it is true. But your heart is the problem. You do not believe in Qi Gong with your full heart."

For the remainder of the day I felt a hollow spot in my chest. I was someone who had seen the truth but still could not totally believe, and my heart sank terribly because of it. I sat in the treatment room and watched as Master Kwan treated patients. Most of these were people who had gone to the hospitals and doctors of Canton and were still sick. They were now trying Master Kwan as a last resort. Like all healers, Master Kwan wished that people would come to see him early in their illness rather than so late. "Coming to see a doctor when you are very sick is like waiting until you are thirsty to dig a well," he said.

Still he accepted all patients. If they were willing to make the climb, then Master Kwan would see them and do his best. No matter who the patients were, when they came to the cave for treatment they were treated equally.

"A patient is just a patient," said Master Kwan. "Look beyond wealth, fame, fortune, power, disgrace, and hardship. Treat them all with the same sense of love and compassion. Only think about alleviating the patient's pain."

It was a sort of Hippocratic oath of Qi Gong.

I sat with the other students and watched as he treated patients. As they came into the cave's entrance, Master Kwan could tell what was wrong with them. For the ones who had never experienced remote diagnosis, it was a jolt. They would look at us and ask how he had known what was wrong with them. For the ones who had been there before, his ability to "see" illness was nothing new. They were amused by the startled looks on the faces of the newcomers.

Once he diagnosed the illness, his treatments began with external Qi. If the problem was a blocked meridian, he would hold his fingers on either side and draw Qi through it. If the problem was something like a tumor, he would point his fingers at it and shoot Qi directly into it. Years later, when I could do this successfully myself, I described it as "radiation, Qi Gong style." Back then, I found these metaphysical aspects of Qi to be very strange. It certainly was not covered anywhere in my medical training at the Military Medical College.

Next, Master Kwan would move to the physical. No matter what the illness, the patients were given Qi Gong exercises that would allow them to direct their own Qi. This was important for two reasons. One was that these exercises worked to boost the Qi energy that he had given them. The other was that the exercises gave the patients an effective means of coping with their own illness.

"It is important that the patients are in control of their health," said Master Kwan. "If they don't feel in control, they will not get well as fast."

If necessary, he would then have an apprentice prepare an herbal remedy from the racks of herbs stored near the cave entrance. Herbs are the backbone of traditional Chinese medicine. Since the days of the Yellow Emperor, three thousand years ago, the Chinese have made healing potions from the bounty of nature. They did not ask why herbs worked in those early days; they just knew certain ones healed certain illnesses. As one Western scholar (Remi Mathieu, *Classic of Mountain and Sea*) noted, the early Chinese had "an understanding of things of nature which seems to compensate for an ignorance of the nature of things."

On this particular day, Master Kwan saw maybe twenty patients. It was the usual parade, ranging from patients with ordinary illnesses to those who left us students wondering why they were still alive.

When one of these very sick patients arrived, Master Kwan would talk to us for a few minutes about his or her case. He had us gather around the patient and listen as he recounted his search for health.

As usual these were fascinating stories. One in particular, however, caught my attention. He was a man of about fifty with a broad smile on his face and black-rimmed glasses that were thick and made his eyes look larger than they were.

He spoke with a slightly hoarse voice but emphasized that he was lucky to be speaking at all. He had the misfortune of having had a tumor on his vocal cords. At first the tumor was small and bothered him only slightly. Then it began to grow until it almost completely stopped his ability to speak. He had been going to a doctor through this period and was finally told that surgery would have to be performed to remove the tumor as well as his vocal cords.

"Of course I didn't want that," said the smiling man. "I would never be able to talk again if that happened. So I came to see Master Kwan."

Master Kwan launched a full attack on the tumor. He administered lengthy sessions of external Qi and gave the man Qi Gong exercises that would improve the flow of his own internal Qi. He also gave him herbal remedies, which the man downplayed, since his other doctors had given him herbs, too, with no results.

"Now the tumor is shrinking," he said. "My doctors in Canton are very happy because they did not want to take away my voice but they thought they had to. Maybe this man can make the tumor go away!"

Master Kwan patted the man on the shoulder and then started his external Qi treatment.

At the end of the day, Master Kwan stood very erect and looked directly at me. The other students knew that his comments were intended for me and they moved slightly away from me as if to avoid the uncomfortable blast of bad energy that was sure to accompany his tirade. He spoke quietly.

"As you can see from watching today's patients, Qi Gong is a science, but a science that has not yet been discovered. It works, it has a system, and its effects can be observed. But they can only be observed if you open your eyes as well as your heart."

3

Gong Fu

After almost a year of traveling to Master Kwan's cave, I felt I had learned very little. Although my housecleaning abilities had improved greatly, I was still just an observer in the healing arts of Qi Gong. I was able to watch Master Kwan as he worked with patients, but I was not taught specific healing techniques. My disappointment ran deep.

I decided to get some advice from my mother.

"I think there are some things that you do not understand about Qi Gong," said my mother after I had told her my story. "Since antiquity, the techniques are passed down through the heart by the master. They involve more than just imitating movements. They require gong fu."

"What is gong fu?" I asked.

"It depends on what you are talking about," she said. "In martial arts, for instance, gong fu is power. A martial artist may be able to perform a routine, but if it does not have power behind the moves, it is said to be without gong fu."

I must have looked confused, because my mother gave another example.

"Gong fu can be applied to art, too," she said. "A painting may be nice to look at, but if it lacks a deep and interesting look, it is said to lack gong fu. The same is true of calligraphy. The most technically perfect writing might not be the most interesting. The calligraphy that is imperfect, yet which carries the style of the calligrapher, would be the one with gong fu."

"So do I lack gong fu?" I asked.

"I don't think you lack it," said my mother. "He is just testing your character, integrity, and perseverance to see if your gong fu is strong enough. Gong fu comes from the heart. It means skills that go below the surface."

I let my mother's words settle in for a moment.

"What should I do?" I asked. "Should I quit going to the cave?"

"If you give up, you lose your chance," said my mother. "If it is not your time, gong fu will not be given to you. But there is one thing that is certain: If you want it, you have to go for it with all your heart."

I threw myself into Qi Gong heart and soul. Through family connections I was able to take a leave of absence from the hospital. The head of my department was surprisingly lenient when he learned that I wanted to study Qi Gong. He had read much about emitted Qi and had seen some of it himself and found it to be quite impressive.

Several days before I left, he called me in to talk. I expected an angry rebuke or at least some mocking of Qi Gong. Instead I was offered hot tea and asked to chat.

"I, too, have been interested in Qi Gong," he told me. "I have seen it heal very difficult diseases and I have wondered how something like this could happen."

He stood to signal the end of our conversation. "We cannot afford to ignore treatments like this. Maybe someday we can work together on a medical study of Qi Gong."

With that I left the hospital and prepared for another journey to Canton. I had no way of knowing at the time that I would be involved in many medical studies showing the positive effects of Qi Gong, both alone and mixed with Western-style medicine. I only knew that in a few hours I would board the southbound train to Canton and give it one more try with Master Kwan.

I arrived late at night and went right to bed in the apprentice chamber of the cave. In the morning I arose very early and got dressed so I would make a good impression on the master.

It appeared to work. Master Kwan was surprised to see me. He looked at me twice as he emerged from his bedchamber, and seemed to have a slight smile on his face as he walked into the treatment room.

Still he ignored me for several days. He addressed the apprentices when he needed something done and seemed to not even notice I was there.

Since I was a student and not an apprentice, that was the way it was supposed to be. It bothered me, though. I had a medical education and knew more than any of the apprentices, some of whom were uneducated peasants who must have shown promise and gong fu to Master Kwan. The youngest apprentice was a six-year-old boy who would someday become a powerful and intelligent Qi Gong master. The oldest apprentice was a seventy-nine-year-old man who had been healed of cancer by Master Kwan and now wanted to understand everything possible about the force that had healed him.

Even as a medical doctor I was inferior to the apprentices

while at the cave. They were, after all, apprentices, while I was only a student.

This time, though, I decided to show none of my previous arrogance about being a doctor. Instead I was respectful and pleasant, even when it hurt.

This time I spent very little time doing cave work. Once the apprentices realized my change in attitude, they spread the cleaning duties more equitably among the students. This gave me more time to watch Master Kwan in action. Much of what I saw I will never forget.

One of the most interesting cases during this time involved not the healing of a human, but of a cow.

It happened this way: Master Kwan and I came down from the mountain one day to go to the market. As we were purchasing vegetables at an outdoor stand, a woman ran through the crowd and stood before Master Kwan.

"Please help us," she begged. "Our cow is sick and needs help."

A sick cow can be a very serious dilemma for rural people in China. Not only do cows provide much-needed milk, but they also plow the fields that keep a family fed and prosperous. Losing a cow can be like losing one's fortune. Because of that, Master Kwan took this woman's concern very seriously.

He followed her to the place where the cow was sitting on a bed of hay. Master Kwan could tell the cow's leg was broken, possibly from stepping into a hole in the field.

With the care that he would show to a human patient, Master Kwan used his external Qi to charge this cow's leg with energy. Then he had the woman and her family splint the animal's leg and gave them instructions on how to care for it.

After a few hours we left and went back to town to continue our shopping. As we walked toward the vegetable stall where the woman had first approached us, Master Kwan stopped and headed instead for an herb shop.

"I must buy some medicine to help the cow," said the master. "That family will lose all of its wealth if the cow does not get well soon."

That night he mixed even more herbs in the cave and sent one of the students in the morning to deliver them to the family. About two weeks later the farmer who owned the cow came up to the cave with baskets of food, including vegetables and freshly slaughtered chickens. The cow was now well and working again, and the farmer wanted to show his gratitude by heaping farm products on Master Kwan.

Gradually, Master Kwan saw a change in me, and when that happened I began to climb the ladder of learning. He began to single me out and explain just what was going on with different patients. At times like this, when he was before a patient, Master Kwan was very quiet, almost subdued. It was at these times that he was most powerful. He would explain to me in careful detail the patient's problem. He would tell me what to look for in conducting my own remote diagnosis, and explain how to see the energy fields that surround us all. He showed me the proper paths of this energy and explained what happened when the energy was blocked or flowing wrong. Then he would show me how to administer external treatments to affect the flow of Qi.

I was still a new student and many of the things I saw left me gaping in wonder.

One woman, for instance, came in with post-polio syndrome. She was a lovely person who had had polio as a child. Now that she was in her late forties, the polio virus had come back to wreak havoc a second time.

She was in considerable pain and was desperate for relief. She had tried Western medicine and even some Chinese techniques like acupuncture, but did not get much relief. Now she decided to come to Master Kwan.

"Why do I always get the patient after everything else has failed?" he joked with the woman.

He had her stand up and turn her back to him. She had serious pain in her left arm and leg, particularly in the foot. Coming up the mountain had left her very tired and I had no doubt that she would rather be sitting than standing for treatment.

"Close your eyes and concentrate on your body," Master Kwan told the woman. "If you start to fall over, don't worry, I am here to catch you."

Master Kwan became very intense. He held his right hand about six inches above her head and pointed the fingers of his left hand at her left arm. He did not touch her, and since her eyes were closed she had no idea what he was doing.

Suddenly her left arm began to quiver. It was subtle at first, but then it began to shake very rapidly as though she were extremely cold.

I looked at the master, but he paid me no heed. With his right hand still above the woman's head, he began to move his left hand down her leg, still not touching it. The leg, too, began to tremble.

I looked at her face. She was perspiring and beads of sweat were forming on her forehead. The lines of tension that she had worn when she arrived were gone, and she was now smiling a sort of blissful smile. Suddenly she began to laugh. At first she emitted just a chuckle, but soon she was laughing uncontrollably.

"I am sorry, Master," she said. "I don't know what is happening. I can't help it."

"That is okay," he told the woman. "If the treatments are working well, many people feel like laughing or crying. Either one is acceptable to me."

After several more minutes of this treatment he had her sit

down so he could work on her foot. She was perspiring greatly now and was no longer self-conscious about laughing. As her foot quivered from the external Qi treatments, she sweated and laughed. Soon everyone in the treatment room was laughing, including the students.

"I must be emitting laughing Qi," said Master Kwan. "That is good medicine, too."

For the next year I climbed the ladder of knowledge. I was at Master Kwan's side at every opportunity. I tried to make the journey to Canton at least twice a month. Almost as often, though, Master Kwan found himself in Shanghai. He was now in great demand among government officials and was constantly being summoned by them. The irony did not escape him.

"Isn't it strange that the people who wanted to put me in jail now want me to make them well?" he asked.

He could have stayed at the best hotels in Shanghai, but chose instead to stay at my mother's house. It was there that I learned some of my best lessons.

One case that stands out in my mind was a provincial governor who had had a stroke and called on Master Kwan to help him. His secretary had called our house and ordered Master Kwan to come to the governor's office.

"Can the governor walk?" asked Master Kwan. When he was told that he could, the master said: "Then have him come here. If he wants to be healed, he must make the effort."

When the governor arrived, we could see that the effort it took to get there had been great. He shuffled into the house, helped by a bodyguard on each arm. By the time he reached the chair that Master Kwan had set up in the middle of the room, the governor was perspiring.

Master Kwan went right to work. He put the governor's feet into a pan of warm water and a damp towel on his head.

The purpose of this was to intensify the power of the Qi that the master began to charge into different parts of the governor's body. Years later, a documentary film was made of Qi Gong in which a master was filmed as he emitted external Qi into the electrodes of an oscilloscope. The charge that he emitted showed up on the scope and looked like jagged mountain peaks across the green screen. Such a charge was now going into the governor, only it was made stronger by the presence of the water.

After twenty minutes of charging the governor with external Qi, Master Kwan stepped back and announced that the treatment was finished.

"Now you must lift your left arm," said the master.

"My arm will not lift," insisted the governor.

"Raise it," demanded Master Kwan. A bodyguard stepped forward to help the governor, but the master waved him away. "Raise it!"

And the governor did. He held his formerly limp hand in front of him and moved the fingers. Then he stood up and stepped out of the pan of water. His legs were now functioning so well that he could walk around the room without assistance.

He walked to a mirror that hung in our hall and looked at his face. Despite the fact that his limbs were now functioning very well, his face still drooped on one side.

"Fix my face," he begged.

Master Kwan shook his head. "I cannot do everything at once," he insisted. "You need more work. You need to come back again and again."

He then gave the governor exercises to improve the function of his limbs and wrote out an herbal prescription.

I was at Master Kwan's cave when he made me an apprentice.

Becoming an apprentice to a Qi Gong master is like becoming an intern after going through medical school. Not only does it signify that you have been learning your lessons adequately, but it represents a major step forward in the way you are trained. Rather than just being able to watch as the master does treatments, you now become a part of the treatment process. To become an apprentice means that you have moved up the ladder that leads to becoming a master. You are with the master at all times and are told all of the techniques and secrets of the healing art. It is truly an honor.

One would then think that the apprentice ceremony would be a solemn event, surrounded by a certain amount of pomp and circumstance. This, however, is not the way it was at all.

Here is how I became an apprentice.

I had been on the mountain for three days on this particular trip. It was my third year of following Master Kwan and I had become more relaxed about my frenetic routine. My bosses at the hospital had now accepted the fact that I was devoted to learning Qi Gong and weaving it into Western medicine, and they had become more tolerant of my absences.

"If each form of medicine is powerful in its own right," I told the chairman of my department, "then both of them together will be even more powerful."

All of the other doctors I worked with had heard my stories and were beginning to believe that Qi Gong was indeed a powerful tool that they could use as well. Informally we made plans to conduct some medical studies on the effects of Qi Gong on cancer patients who were undergoing chemotherapy. We wanted to see if Qi treatments increased the healing effects of the chemo.

My life had settled down as a result of this acceptance.

Now I was standing at the mouth of the cave, savoring a moment of true inner peace. I remember well being taken by the beauty of the hazy mountain peaks in the distance and the fresh morning air. The air was cool to the lungs, and I closed my eyes and began to draw in a deep chestful.

Suddenly there was a crushing blow to the top of my head. For a moment I thought a rock had fallen from the ceiling. I groped for balance and struggled to open my eyes. When they opened, all I could see was a universe of stars racing across my field of vision.

I felt my way to a boulder and leaned against it. As I cradled my head in my hands, Master Kwan stepped next to me.

"It is done now," he said seriously. "You are an apprentice."

"You did that?" I asked.

"I had to," he said. "It is done that way. Now you are an apprentice. This signifies its beginning."

As I held my head, the master continued his explanation.

"There are two major meridian points," he said. "There is the very top of your head and the very bottom of your body, that area called the perineum. When I hit you like that I awakened your spirit with energy. The only way your spirit can be awakened is when a master puts his energy into this meridian in this way. Congratulations. You are now an apprentice."

Later that day, Master Kwan performed other rituals that I have been sworn never to tell. I can say that these are secret rituals handed down through the ages. They are known by few people, yet they have affected the health of millions worldwide.

He did, however, offer other information about the ability to heal that I can write about because it provides an understanding of how we can all tap the mysterious forces of healing that are available to every one of us.

These forces, said Master Kwan, come from the heart and the subconscious. Some people can muster these forces at will, which gives them a high level of mastery over the energy in the universe.

Sometimes people who have faced trauma are adept at tapping into this energy. This is particularly true of those who have died and then come back, especially those who have had near-death experiences that put them in touch with departed loved ones or with higher spirit beings. These people are often blessed with special powers after their experiences, and sometimes those powers involve the ability to heal.

Prayer and meditation can also put us in touch with the forces of healing, said Master Kwan. The reason for this is simple: Deep relaxation can release one's preconceived notions about life and allow one to enter into a state of universal wholeness.

"Stress, suppression, and pain are all psychological states that induce physiological changes," said Master Kwan. "Yet spirit, soul, courage, and ambitions are all a part of psychology, too, but they are generally pressed down into the subconscious mind. This area of the brain can be opened and its contents used if we just achieve deep relaxation."

For an apprentice to become a master, he or she must learn how to tap into this universal healing energy. The best way to do that, said Master Kwan, is through Qi Gong exercises. I have found this to be true. Over the years I have found that Qi and blood are inseparable in that they are practically the same thing. The best way to control them both is through exercises that lead to mystical enlightenment.

The backbone of early Taoism was the secret of longevity. It was the belief of the ancient followers of this religion, as it is today, that one had to practice sacred physical and breathing exercises, eat a good diet, and be knowledgeable in the arts of herbal medicine before one could become a candidate for immortality.

The exercises practiced by the ancients are represented on silk paintings found in ancient tombs. The paintings are of men and women performing these exercises. Along with these methods there are written specific therapeutic benefits, such as positions to alleviate knee pain or numbness or even deafness.

These early forms of Qi Gong were called *daoyin* exercises and were explained this way by an ancient physician in the *Zhuangzi*, an early medical journal: "Whoever exhales and inhales, breathing vigorously and calmly, who expels stale air and imbibes fresh air, who suspends one's self like a bear and stretches out one's limbs like a bird, is seeking none other than longevity. Such is the ideal of those who cultivate their bodies by stretching and contracting."

Over the next several days, Master Kwan taught me a series of these exercises, a grouping of eight Qi Gong exercises. I have modified them over the years, and call them the Golden Eight.

Regardless of the weather, I arose at dawn and did these exercises over and over for at least two hours each day. In driving rain I found protection under which to work out. During the hot season I took off clothing, and when I was in a cold climate I put on clothing. Even if I had stayed up late the night before, I would arise in the early-morning hours and do this painstakingly deliberate routine nonstop for at least two hours.

The purpose of these exercises is to put one in touch with the unconscious mind, or, as Master Kwan said, "to make conscious the unconscious." To do that, one must focus on such aspects of oneself as the mind, form, and breath. It is only through this type of focus that one can truly achieve the sort of intensity necessary to becoming a master.

Doing these exercises was never easy. Sometimes I would start the day thinking that maybe I would cut the routine short just this one time and go back to bed. After all, who would know? The answer to that question was obvious: I would know. If anything, I knew that the path to mastery led to an understanding of myself. If I skipped a routine or cut it short, I would only be fooling myself. I now understood the Chinese proverb "A master must eat bitters every day," because every day was hard.

"This seems like an extremely difficult way to become a master," I said one night to Master Kwan as we sat with the other apprentices in the cave's examining room. "I feel like people are watching me and expecting great things. How long will it take?"

"It takes time," said Master Kwan. "When it happens, though, people will marvel."

"Then it will be worth the effort," I said.

"Yes," said Master Kwan, "just like the story 'How Yu Gong Moved the Mountain.' Do you remember that? Yu Gong was a man who realized that if he could move a mountain, then he would have a larger field on which to grow crops. He told his friends about this and they laughed at him. 'No one can move a mountain with just one shovel and a bucket,' they declared. Still Yu Gong started digging and moving soil. Eventually he moved the mountain and became very rich from the crops. So you see, everything can be done if you do it just a shovelful at a time."

The Taoists said, "That which is above is the same as that which is below," and "The microcosm reflects the macrocosm." This means that we as human beings should be as orderly in our lives as is the behavior of the planets and the stars in the universe.

When I did these exercises so intensely, I felt completely

at harmony with myself and the world around me. Taoists believe that most disease is caused by stress and anxiety, two conditions that keep the organs from functioning properly. In the two hours a day that I did these exercises, I was free of tension and lost in the universe. Even though I was sore and uninspired when I started them, I was sweating and filled with Qi when I finished. That is the way it was.

I had an opportunity to work more closely with Master Kwan during this period and to even have some patients of my own. I also experienced more of Master Kwan's super-conscious abilities.

One time, for instance, Master Kwan sent me to treat a patient in Chuansha, a seacoast town near Shanghai. This man was in charge of all of the seafood that came into this city, which meant that every fish that was caught by a commercial fisherman had to be accounted for by this man's office. As you can imagine, this was a big job.

"No wonder he is sick," said a friend when I told him where I was going. "Anyone responsible for that much math is bound to be sick."

In some ways that was true. This man's problem was hypertension. His duties were so stressful that he was constantly worried. He not only had to make sure that the fish were counted but that they were shipped to market quickly. All of this pressure from the outside had created high blood pressure on the inside.

He had taken blood pressure medication, but it left him feeling light-headed, which increased his tension even more. Now he was not only worried about his high blood pressure, but he was afraid that he might black out at work, which would lead to rumors about his competence.

A friend told him that Qi Gong could help his blood pressure without medication, and mentioned Master Kwan.

Word went out through the grapevine, and before long I was contacted by Master Kwan at the hospital in Shanghai. He was in town, but he was busy treating a government official and could not make the short trip to Chuansha.

"I would do it myself, but this is not a big problem," said the master. "It is fairly easy. If it is just normal hypertension, teach him the appropriate exercises."

I was well versed in the treatment of hypertension. Recent experiments conducted by a number of medical colleges in China had shown that Qi Gong exercises alone were highly effective in treating high blood pressure. I had seen Master Kwan treat many patients with this disease and knew essentially what to do.

I borrowed a motorcycle and rode the fifty miles to Chuansha. The fish manager was glad to see me. He took me into his office and locked the door. For the next hour I showed him a number of exercises that would help him overcome his problem.

He learned quickly and I was quite proud of myself. There was one problem, however. I was now finding it possible to see the meridians like Master Kwan did during his remote diagnosis. When I first examined the fish manager I noticed that his kidney meridian was blocked. Rather than treat that as well, I decided to see if the exercises alone would be enough.

The fish manager was so grateful for the treatment that he ordered an entire truck to be loaded with yellow fin crocker and driven to my house. In all there must have been five hundred pounds of fish following me as I rode home on the motorcycle. We were able to keep some of the fish in my mother's refrigerator, but most of it had to be stored in a freezer at the hospital.

After the truck driver and I unloaded the fish, I began to feel guilty. Since I did not open the kidney meridian, I felt as though I had treated only half of the fish manager's problem. His high blood pressure would certainly be lowered by the exercises I had given him, but the only way there would be a permanent effect would be if I treated the blocked kidney meridian. The reason I had not done so was that I was not sure about the treatment and I was too proud to call Master Kwan. Now I felt embarrassed.

I went back to my mother's house and telephoned Master Kwan at the home where he was staying. When he came to the telephone he was laughing.

"You get the gift, but I have to do the healing," he said.

"How did you know?" I asked.

"A Qi Gong master knows what is bothering his apprentices even before they tell him," he said. "That is part of my gong fu."

I told him what I had seen when I did my remote diagnosis of the fish manager. He said that my hunch was right, that there were three more meridians blocked. He told me where to administer external Qi to unblock them and offered an herbal prescription for me to concoct if the blockages did not go away.

"You must go back to him in the morning and complete the treatment," said Master Kwan. "It is important to be as thorough as possible."

I experienced Master Kwan's extranormal abilities many other times as well.

Once Master Kwan took me to the distant town of Yi-Hsien, known internationally for its tea utensils made from purple sand. These are priceless works of art, made by very skilled artisans, and the master was called to treat one of the best of these artists for an illness. He treated this man successfully, and soon he was feeling well and working again. To show his gratitude, the artist asked me to carry three of his beautiful tea sets to Master Kwan.

As I carried these back to the master at a local hotel where we were staying, I began to think that I would like one of these sets for myself. Why not? I had helped with the treatments, too, and besides, there were still two left for the master. I took one to my room and then carried the other two to the master.

When I set them on the table, he looked curiously at them. "Only two?" he asked.

"Yes," I said. "Only two."

Later that evening I began to feel sick to my stomach. I did some Qi Gong exercises, but they did no good. I drank green tea and massaged my stomach, but that did no good, either. As I sat on the floor, perspiring and in pain, I focused on the table on which the tea set was sitting.

"That is it," I said. "That is what is causing it."

I picked up the tea set and carried it to the master's room. When he answered the door, I told him about my error in judgment and asked for his forgiveness.

The master invited me in and asked me to sit down. I thought he would be angry, but in fact he was pleased that I had returned the tea set, and took credit for my excruciating stomach pain.

"Now you know why I asked you if there were only two tea sets," he said. "You showed no remorse, so I gave you the pain to teach you that to live the life of man, a man must be upstanding, honest, and have integrity. Man always has thoughts of dishonesty, but you must learn to ignore them."

At that moment, the pain in my stomach went away.

Becoming a master requires adherence to a set of rules that has been handed down for thousands of years. A true master is in touch with the balance of nature. As Master Kwan said: "The universe's energy is equal and just. When evil arises, the universal forces of balance will be exerted naturally. As an apprentice you must remember the traditional Chinese culture and laws. Qi Gong calls for respect of all things and all people, including your master and the Tao, 'the way.'

"I myself remember these cultures and rules and live by them. What you have learned through your master is yours. Your master will always treat you like a son and you must always respect him like a father. It is through this kind of respect that Qi Gong has survived through generations of war, turmoil, and changing dynasties. That is the way Qi Gong lives on."

I witnessed this almost clannish devotion on the day that the grand master came from the mountains of Hunan to visit Master Kwan. All of the apprentices were told to line up like soldiers and to stand very straight as the grand master visited. That is just what we did. No one dared to speak to "Master's Master," and he did not speak to us. We watched and listened as the two men spoke, and felt very lucky just to be there.

To the world outside this seems very formal. But to the world of Qi Gong this was the way it was. As I tell my students now: "There is a rule of the ladder that applies to Qi Gong. The master is above you on the ladder and he looks down on you until you are educated enough to look him in the eye."

I now understand the rule of the ladder. As an apprentice, though, I thought I was not subject to this rule until I got knocked down a rung or two.

4

The Chosen

Once I became an apprentice, Master Kwan became very harsh with me. If I made a mistake in treating someone, he was quick to reprimand me in front of the patient and then take over the treatment. This was always embarrassing, since it lowered my standing with the patient as well as my opinion of myself.

The other apprentices had a different view of the master's harshness. They thought it meant good news for me.

"He obviously favors you over us," said Apprentice Wang. "He will not allow you to make even the smallest mistake. He does not treat the rest of us like that. I think he expects mistakes from us. You are the chosen one."

Still I was not happy with this type of treatment. One time, after being humiliated in front of a patient, I asked Master Kwan why he was so inflexible toward me.

"Because you have the highest education of everyone here," he said. "I want you to introduce Qi Gong to the world of Western medicine. That can only be done through a doctor. I want you to be able to explain it using Western medical terms. This is a science that has not yet been explored and it will be up to you to explore it."

What he said was certainly true. Although the other apprentices were quite talented, they were largely peasants, bureaucrats, and soldiers. Although some of them had degrees in higher education, none of them had any formal training in medical science. A few of them could not even read.

"He has made you the seed apprentice," said Wang. "You are the one who is supposed to go out and spread this knowledge to the medical community so they will start using it. Congratulations."

Congratulations, indeed. Eventually I would be glad to have had such a tough taskmaster. At the time, however, I did not feel like the chosen one. Rather, I felt like the one who had been singled out for punishment.

For instance, I was severely punished for taking notes. Note taking had always been taboo in the world of Qi Gong, anyway. In ancient times, Qi Gong masters were feared for their powers by members of the upper class, who sometimes sought them out and killed them. Since notes could serve as proof that a person had studied Qi Gong, they were abolished by the masters of this healing art. Those who studied Qi Gong became a sort of secret society, with information being passed down by word of mouth.

Over the years, this need to be secret diminished. Books were written on Qi Gong, and its masters became celebrities who received as much awe and respect as high government officials. This idolatry to those outside of the government alarmed Mao Ze-dong, who wanted all people to be treated the same (except those in government, of course). He ordered prison sentences for those who dared practice Qi Gong and other forms of traditional healing. It was during this period that Master Kwan was sent to jail, where he undoubtedly cursed every note and book about Qi Gong that the Red Guard had found in his home. It was at that point that some of his negative feelings about note taking were formed.

Master Kwan's edict against notes presented a problem for me. I had always been an avid note taker. I took such copious notes through school that one of the teachers jokingly said that I was trying to rewrite the textbooks. In medical school I was such an avid note taker that fellow students who had missed class would always ask me if they could borrow my notes so they could catch up with the rest of us. Yet in working with Master Kwan I was told to take no notes. "Commit it to memory," he said. "That is the only way to become a master."

"You don't understand," I said. "The way I commit it to memory is by writing it down."

"No, it is you who do not understand," said Master Kwan. "Look at these other apprentices. Some of them cannot even read, yet they work very hard to learn things without even being able to read. The way you commit things to memory is by working very hard and paying attention!"

I could not argue with that. Through struggle and hard work, the other apprentices had learned their lessons very well. Not one of them ever took notes. All they did was watch and learn. But I had a different learning process than they did. Long after everyone had gone to bed, I sat up in the examining room and took notes about the patients we had seen that day and the treatments we had used to effect healing.

Because I stayed up so late, I sometimes slept in late in the morning. There were many occasions on which the other apprentices had awakened early and done all of the cave work before I got up. I was not doing this intentionally; I was just staying up much later than the others, and therefore could not get up with them. My tardiness on these mornings infuriated Master Kwan. On these days he would tell me to practice my exercises longer and be even harsher with me than usual.

One day I was treating a patient for insomnia when the master rudely interrupted me and took over the treatment. I was very angry, but I stood quietly at his side until he was finished with the patient. Then I asked him what I had done wrong.

"Your heart is not in it," he said. "You have to use your heart to learn it. What you are doing is taking notes so you can somehow explain it to yourself. Let it flow through your heart instead of your brain. Do not intellectualize it or you will become confused. You will try to apply the rules of logic to Qi Gong, which you cannot really do until you learn how to do Qi Gong."

I understood what Master Kwan was saying, but I did not want to do it. I had a certain way of learning, and taking notes was part of it. I was completely inflexible on that matter.

Unfortunately, so was Master Kwan.

One day, as I took notes, an apprentice tapped on my shoulder. "Master wants to see you," he said.

I put my notebook down and followed him outside. There, by one of the side entrances to the cave, was a wooden crate that was maybe five feet tall. Sitting around it with nervous looks on their faces were the other apprentices. Master Kwan stood in front of it with a stern look on his face.

"I have asked you many times to stop taking notes and learn by example," he said, with a fiery look in his eyes. "Now *you* will become an example. Please get in the box."

He held open a door to reveal what was inside. Nails had been pounded through the top and penetrated a few inches into the box. On the floor of the box was a pile of burning incense.

"Get in," he said. Without argument I did what I was told. It was extremely uncomfortable. I could not sit down because the incense would burn my rear end. Yet I could not stand fully, either, without the nails poking me in the head. I just hunched over and watched with despair as Master Kwan closed the door.

"Now you will listen to me," he said to me through the air holes. "Now you will know that I mean what I say."

I spent several hours in this wooden prison, perspiring heavily and breathing the scented smoke from the incense. Standing in this crumpled position for so long left me exhausted. By the time someone opened the door, I was barely able to straighten up, and my feet were so cramped that I am sure the stint in the box is a main reason my feet are so strong today.

As I walked inside the cave to eat lunch, the other apprentices cleared a place for me to sit down. They were talkative and chattered to one another freely as I sat in silence. It was hard for me to put my feelings together after spending time in the box. On one hand I felt as though I had been made a fool of, while on the other hand I felt as though I had been elevated another rung on the ladder. Either way, I understood that I would now be learning without notes.

Any anger I had over the box incident subsided as I began to spend more time with Master Kwan and his patients. As usual there were many miracles.

Late one night, for instance, we heard a group of people come into the cave's entrance. When people arrived this late, they would usually find a comfortable place to spread a blanket and sleep until morning when everyone got up. But these people had no intentions of doing that. They came into the mouth of the cave and began to shout for help.

A few of the apprentices, including myself, got out of bed

to see what was going on. In the middle of the patient room were a man in a stretcher, the four people who had carried him, and his wife. She was a wiry and energetic woman who carried two baskets, one filled with oranges and the other with eggs.

She said hello to everyone but did not tell us why they had come until Master Kwan came into the room. He had obviously been sleeping soundly and looked tired, as though he had walked into a dream.

The woman approached him and with a worried look on her face gave him the oranges and eggs as advance payment for the healing she hoped would take place.

Master Kwan handed the baskets to an apprentice and approached the man on the stretcher. He was a slender man with a look of both concern and pain on his face. He wore an official-looking uniform of some kind and had his right foot heavily bandaged.

"Tell me the story," said Master Kwan.

"My husband is a security guard," said the woman, stepping forward. "He saw a thief on the roof of the business where he works and climbed up to capture him. The man started to run away and my husband followed him. As he started to run, he slipped on the roof and fell off. He has broken his ankle in three places."

The man had immediately been taken to a hospital, where X rays of the foot showed three fractures. The doctors wanted to perform an operation that would pin the bones together, but it cost so much money that it would take the family years to pay it back. Desperate for a solution they could afford, the woman convinced her neighbors to carry her husband up the mountain to see Master Kwan. "Although it is late," said the woman, "I knew you would not mind an emergency call."

The woman was right; Master Kwan did not seem to mind

the intrusion at all. He turned to one apprentice and told him to go get a bottle of rice wine and a bowl. He positioned the man in the middle of the room and poured wine into the bowl. Then he put some wine into his mouth and sprayed the man's feet with alcohol. Three times he did this before setting the bowl down and charging the man's foot with external Qi. When he did this, the man's foot began to twitch as though the muscles were cramping. The man looked terrified at first, as his muscles tightened. Then his face relaxed as the pain subsided. Soon he was almost giddy and claimed that his foot felt as though it were being tickled by the master.

"Get up," said Master Kwan.

With no hesitation, the man stood up and began to walk. He was happy at being able to walk, but his foot still had a substantial amount of pain when he put weight on it.

"Try this," said the master. He held his hand over a cup of hot tea and charged it with his Qi. Then he handed it to the man and told him to drink it as fast as possible.

"I can feel it in my foot," said the man excitedly. He began to walk with greater ease now and everyone in his party was extremely happy.

Master Kwan was not finished yet. He went to a medicine box and pulled out a number of herbs. Then he ground them with a mortar and pestle and moistened them to make a poultice for the bruised area of the man's foot. Packing it on the foot, he wrapped it with clean cloth and declared the man on the road to recovery.

When he was finished, the man's wife and the neighbors who had brought him up the mountain all bowed.

"You are a great healer," announced the wife.

"I am a *tired* great healer," said Master Kwan, bowing and going back to his bedroom.

For him it was all in a day's work. For me and the other apprentices it was a marvel.

I was now seeing many such successes with patients, inspiring me even further. I put the humiliation of the box incident aside and began to listen closely to every word that the master said. If seeing is believing, then I was now a true believer, opening my heart to the lessons of the master.

My sincerity must have shown through, because Master Kwan began to treat me differently. Rather than treat me like a truculent pupil, he now treated me like a son.

"Now it is time for you to climb higher up the ladder," he told me one day. "From now on you will be a different person."

He then gave me the rules by which I would have to live.

"For the next one hundred days you must practice harder than you have ever practiced before. I will give you secret exercises for building your ability to emit external Qi. They are unwritten, and are passed down only through the masters. Do not reveal them to anyone else or you will lose your power."

I was to practice these exercises every available minute of each day. Master Kwan even said that I should do these exercises during my meal breaks at the hospital instead of eating. When I protested, he said simply, "Think of them as food of a different kind."

When I looked at him with curiosity, he patiently explained.

"Buddhists are known for their techniques of spiritual development," he said. "But we are Taoists and are more practical than Buddhists. We emphasize the importance of developing both the physical and the spiritual aspects of life, while at the same time building enlightenment.

"That is why the physical conditioning is so important, especially in the beginning. But our form of conditioning is different from the modern conceptions of conditioning like distance running or strength training. Rather, it utilizes Qi

Gong techniques to control breathing, thoughts, and physical form.

"These exercises entail the extremes of life. When you do them, you will see that there is passiveness within activeness; activeness within passiveness, *extreme* passiveness generating activeness, and *extreme* activeness generating passiveness. These exercises are sometimes both yin and yang at the same time. This way, you can reach a complete harmony of body and soul that helps the physical body reach a greater state of enlightenment."

The next one hundred days held other surprises for me as well. "You can have no sex at all during this time," said Master Kwan, a slight smile on his face. "Abstaining from sex will open your meridians and increase your energy. During the last thirty days you will understand. Your energy will build and become greater than it has ever been before."

I tried not to look as though this abstinence would be a burden. I smiled shyly and said that if things got too bad, maybe I could relax with a glass of wine.

"That is another thing," said Master Kwan. "You can never drink again. When we have alcohol in our bodies, we lose control of our Qi. Sometimes it runs wild, and at other times it drops very low. Because of that, people throughout history have made terrible mistakes as a result of drinking liquor. A Qi Gong master must never drink liquor because he must always be in control of his senses."

Giving up alcohol would not be a problem for me. I had never been very fond of spirits anyway, and we certainly never had any alcohol at home—where my mother referred to it as "the devil in a bottle." Alcohol had a bad reputation in China and was most certainly responsible for the fall of at least one dynasty. I was well educated in the evils of alcohol and felt no sense of loss at being forbidden to imbibe anymore.

"Then there is one other thing," said Master Kwan. "You must not be greedy for money. I know that you need money to survive. But it must not be the reason that you treat someone. A peasant gets the same treatment as an emperor. If you break these rules, your power will drop."

From this point on, Master Kwan kept me close. He became more of a teacher and less of a taskmaster. He watched as I worked with patients and was not so harsh when I made mistakes.

When I was in Shanghai, the master would frequently drop in at the hospital. He had a high opinion of Western-style medicine and always expressed his belief that a patient must do what is best for the patient, and not what is best for the doctor.

"Some doctors don't like it when I see their patients," he told me. "Patients come to me and say they want to keep their visit to a Qi Gong master secret from their doctor. I say, 'What's the big deal? It is your body, isn't it? Make up your own mind.'"

Although he had respect for Western medicine and was impressed by the enormous size of its hospitals, he felt that most of the medical equipment used was unnecessary. One day I showed him an X-ray machine, thinking he would be impressed by its ability to look inside the human body. When I held up a film and showed him the pictures we had taken with it, he just shook his head.

"This is a waste of time and money," he said. "I can do the same thing by just looking at a patient. Maybe more doctors should study Qi Gong and then they would not have to buy these machines."

Of course I did not agree with Master Kwan and I still do not. It would be foolish for me to argue that medical technology like X-ray machines and other imaging devices are not effective and important. But it would also be foolish to argue that such technology is infallible. There is always room for error in X-ray results, whether the error is due to the image that is taken or the interpretation of that image by doctors. Master Kwan had one such story in which he beat an imaging machine.

He was contacted by the medical staff of a very high government official who was having problems with his left hand after a stroke. Among other things, his hand strength would sometimes diminish and he had tingling sensations in his forearm. At first these symptoms were just a minor annoyance, but when they became worse, his doctors ordered a battery of X rays and scans to see just what was wrong. They carefully examined the entire pathway to his left hand, by doing CT scans of his brain, spine, shoulders, and so on.

When they could find nothing, they called in Master Kwan.

"It was very simple for me," declared Master Kwan. "I came and sat with this man for a while and could tell by looking at his meridians that there was a tiny spot in his brain that was dead from the stroke. I told them it was on the right side of his brain and told them in which area to look. The next day they did a CT scan, and I was right."

As I began to understand my relationship to Master Kwan, I also understood his relationship to the grand master. When this man visited the cave, I noticed a distinct difference in the way Master Kwan acted. There seemed to be a power shift, in that Master Kwan deferred to this man in the way that I deferred to Master Kwan.

The way this happened was intriguing. Word of the grand master's arrival immediately spread throughout the cave. The apprentices then sprang into action. They offered him the best chair and brought him a cup of tea, both of which he refused. Only when Master Kwan made the offer would the grand master accept it: He would sit only in the chair that was offered by Master Kwan, and drink only the tea that was given to him by his student.

You never quit being someone's student, even as a master. Of course, you always showed respect to your master. You did not sit before the master did, nor did you drink your tea before him. When giving your master tea or food, you always held it with two hands, never one.

When the grand master visited the cave, I stayed as close to him as possible. He had only one eye and I tried to stay on his blind side so he would not notice me as I hovered close to him. I knew that the grand master was there to teach Master Kwan some new techniques, and I also wanted to learn what I could.

I thought I was fooling him by staying on his blind side, but I was wrong. The grand master knew I was there. He was simply ignoring me, said Master Kwan.

"Everything has its stage," said Master Kwan. "In life there are always stages like a stairway. My master knows you are looking over his shoulder, but he is ignoring you. My master will only come down the stairs to teach me. He has no relationship with you, which is why he will never take anything from you. With me it is different. He is my master and will take everything I offer him. That is how the relationship is supposed to be between master and pupil. You cannot run up the stairs and learn. The master comes down the stairs and teaches the pupil and then goes back up. Someday I will come down the stairs and teach you what he has taught me."

By now I had become a spectacle at the hospital. In my private moments I would find a quiet room and practice the Qi-building exercises. Sometimes my colleagues would come into the room and watch me. It made me uncomfortable to know that they were there, but I could not stop doing these Qi Gong exercises just because someone walked in. Instead I would pretend the person was not there and continue to focus on my task.

Soon word began to spread that I was studying advanced Qi Gong. Some of my colleagues were not bothered by what I was doing. They could see the value in Qi Gong and were glad that someone had the courage to mix some traditional Chinese medicine with Western medicine. Some of the other doctors became quite angry and thought I should be reprimanded for practicing Qi Gong in a Western-style hospital.

"Perhaps you should keep your Qi Gong to yourself for a while," said one of my friends.

I agreed, and decided to do something that doctors would not dare do in America. Without telling the patients, I secretly mixed Qi Gong treatments with Western medicine. With some patients, I would give them Western medicine for their problems. With other patients, I would just give them vitamin pills and tell them they were being given powerful medicine. Then I would administer external Qi treatments. The problems I treated in this way included high blood pressure, heart disease, and bone disease. Overall, the patients treated with Qi Gong fared better than those who were treated only with Western medicine.

I thought I was doing this work on the sly, but apparently people noticed what I was doing. As I left the hospital in the evening, people began to approach me and ask if I could help them with their medical problems. Usually I denied that I was treating patients with Qi Gong. One night, however, I was approached by a desperate-looking woman with tears in her eyes.

"My mother is very sick," she said. "The hospital says that she has to get her hip replaced because it has become arthritic. But they now say they cannot do the surgery because she has a bad heart and would die if they operate. They have sent her home with little hope of living. What can you do?"

There was so much desperation in the woman's eyes that I told her I would take a look at her mother. I got the address of her apartment and promised to come the next day.

The entire family had gathered for my arrival. I was escorted into the tiny living room by the woman I had seen the night before. She introduced me to everyone in the room and then led me to one of the apartment's two bedrooms. Lying on a narrow bed was the woman's seventy-seven-year-old mother. She had been trying to take a nap, but was afraid to fall asleep because she thought she might die.

"Ever since the hospital told her she might die during surgery, she has had trouble sleeping," said the daughter. "She also cannot get out of bed."

I had become good at remote diagnosis by now and could tell that this woman was in deep trouble. Her hip joint was getting very little blood, and because of that the joint was seizing up. This was true of the muscles around the joint as well. Her heart disease had progressed to the point that it was affecting circulation in her legs, a condition known in the West as peripheral vascular disease. She very definitely had hip and heart problems, but she also had very strong Qi. She did not want to die.

My approach with this patient would be to improve her circulation using a combination of Qi Gong and herbal remedies. It was the approach I had learned from Master Kwan and it is the approach I have used on virtually every patient since.

Using external Qi treatments, I was able to relax the muscles of her hip. "My goal is to get you out of bed so you can do exercises to make you stronger," I explained to her.

I also put the woman on a special diet that consisted largely of beef broth. To this I had her add herbs that open the arteries and increase circulation.

After a few external Qi treatments over the course of three days, I gave her Chinese herbs aimed at improving the strength of her kidneys and liver, which had become weak and were not performing the duties needed to keep her arteries clear of fat and cholesterol. She was also losing a lot of calcium through her urine, which was decreasing the density of this important mineral in her bones. By strengthening her liver and kidney meridians, I was able to stop the further degeneration of her bones.

Within one week she was able to get out of bed and walk without help from family members. At that point I gave her a number of Qi Gong exercises that she could perform on her own. The physical purpose of these exercises was to unblock meridians and balance her Qi, which, in addition to other things, would build strength in her legs and improve her sense of balance. There was a mental purpose as well: These exercises gave the woman improved confidence and a sense of control over her well-being.

After one month she returned to the hospital for a follow-up examination by her physician. When he saw the woman walk into the examining room, he was surprised. "You are looking better," he exclaimed. The real surprise came, however, when he examined the X rays of her hip. Although there were still signs of scarring, the hip joint was healing. The muscles around the joint were supple and strong and the woman's flexibility was greatly improved.

"How is your heart?" asked the doctor.

"I am walking every day," she said. "I am even challenging it with special exercises that are giving it energy. And I am taking herbs, too."

"Who prescribed all of this for you?" asked the curious doctor.

Although we had agreed that my involvement would be kept secret, the woman was so elated that she let my identity slip. "One of your own people," she said gleefully. "Dr. Hong Liu, who is also a Qi Gong doctor."

5

Qi Gong, M.D.

Word spread after that, and soon I was besieged by patients who wanted Qi Gong healing. I was told that I could not do Qi Gong at the hospital. Even though the Cultural Revolution had ended and traditional treatments were making a comeback in Chinese society, many doctors were still leery about letting anyone practice Qi Gong at an official state institution.

"There are still people who think that the Cultural Revolution was the correct thing to do," said one of the hospital's top doctors. "If they came back into power, we would be severely reprimanded."

This presented a problem for the physicians who ran the hospital, since there were many patients who did not respond to conventional treatment but who would perhaps respond to Qi Gong. Even though they acted like politicians, these doctors were still interested in healing. They were curious about Qi Gong, too, and wanted to see how it would work in a modern hospital setting. It would not be until the 1980s that some of these same doctors would be among those to establish official Qi Gong research laboratories. Now they were willing to let me practice on my own.

"You can take patients, but only if you treat them outside of the hospital," one of the doctors told me. "But please keep us informed about how things work out."

Of course I was elated. Now I did not have to hide my involvement with Qi Gong. It was not official, but it was not unofficial, either. That was as good as it was going to be for a while.

As my first "semi-official" patient I chose a woman with a breast tumor. It was not a cancerous tumor, but one that the doctors thought may someday turn into cancer. I went to her home to treat her.

Her medical report said that it was a fibrous tumor in her left breast, about eight centimeters around. At this point I had never dealt with a tumor alone and I became nervous. What if I make a mistake? I thought. What if I make her worse?

I suddenly became very cautious. After examining the tumor, I told the patient that I would be back in a few days and immediately left for the train station. The next morning, I found myself standing in front of a surprised Master Kwan at the mouth of his cave.

"What is wrong?" he asked. "Are you hiding from somebody?"

He offered me tea in the treatment room and I told him about the situation at the hospital and the woman's tumor.

"I want to be very careful with this case," I said. "I need your help in getting rid of this tumor."

Master Kwan nodded and set down his tea.

"Tumors have a lot of emotion and stress in them," he said. "When people are stressed by their environment or when their family life or love life is bad, they often have liver problems. Once the liver gets a blockage like this, then the body is susceptible to tumors."

"What do I do for that?" I asked.

"Unblock the liver channel and let the bad energy flow out of the body," he said. "That will shrivel the tumor."

Master Kwan gave me a bagful of herbs to enhance the Qi and sent me on my way.

Using external Qi, I worked on the tumor and the blockage of the liver meridian. Then I gave my patient a decoction of the herbs along with a number of Qi Gong exercises for her to perform twice a day.

Within two weeks, the tumor shrank substantially, but it did not disappear. Once again, I was in a quandary about treatment and knew of only one way to get out. Wishing for telephone service, I boarded the southbound train and headed for Master Kwan's cave.

"With this patient, you need to focus more on mental healing," said Master Kwan, as I explained the problem while relaxing in the treatment room after my long journey. "I will give you some new herbs that will increase the circulation of Qi. But you must give her exercises that will make her focus on her mind, spirit, and breathing. That way, she will forget about her emotional problems and focus on killing that tumor."

Once again I returned to Shanghai to treat the woman's tumor. I gave her the herbs and different Qi Gong exercises. This time the results were different. Her tumor virtually disappeared within two weeks. X rays showed only a tiny portion remaining.

The successful treatment of this woman's tumor caused a slight commotion among the doctors on the staff. The ones who were familiar with the woman's case found the before-and-after X rays difficult to believe. After they had the chance to examine her in person, they all wondered how a tumor like this could have disappeared.

s this work?" they asked.

n that I did not entirely understand what was

ce they were all familiar with acupuncture,

....., I drew certain comparisons between the two ancient medical arts.

"Qi circulates throughout the body through a network of twelve channels called meridians," I said. "These are like waterways and they feed nourishment and energy to the different organs of the body. A Qi master can put energy into those meridians in the same way that an acupuncturist can insert a needle. Qi Gong exercises also can put energy into these meridians."

Not only do these exercises and external Qi emissions open meridian channels, they also direct both Qi and blood to the area where the specific illness resides. If Qi were a glowing ball, then the Qi Gong exercises would move that glowing ball along the meridians to the area of the body that needs Qi the most.

A patient with prostate cancer, for instance, would direct healing energy to the prostate gland by doing Qi Gong exercises. He would also relax his entire physical and mental being to such an extent that the Qi would have a concentrated effect upon the disease, perhaps because there would be little stress to interfere with the healing process. It is as Master Kwan had told me: "The moment a patient relaxes and calms his fears, he can feel the energy of the universe in his body. That is when Qi can begin its healing."

With herbal medicines, Qi Gong exercises, and external Qi, healing is quicker and more effective.

Within a few weeks, a doctor told me about one of his patients with cancer. It had started in the patient's lungs and had now spread throughout his entire body. He had come to the hospital late in the diseased state, and the only thing the doctors had to offer was chemotherapy. The man had reject-ed that option.

He had decided to go home and wait for the inevitable. Did I want to see him? asked the doctor. I said that I would and was given the man's address.

A few days later I picked up his files from the hospital and went to his home. He lived in a nice apartment in one of the buildings the French had built during a period of European intervention in China. He greeted me at the door and then shuffled back to the chair where he now spent his days.

His was a difficult case. Lung cancer is a tough problem to treat with any form of medicine. Plus the cancer had spread throughout his body, making the problem greater by a thou-sandfold.

I examined him for a while and then went home to pack my bag. I had to board the train for Canton once again for a consultation with Master Kwan.

At the cave I explained the case to the master. I could see from the concern in his face that he knew this might be beyond the scope of any treatment. He did not tell me that, however. Instead he told me how to conduct my treatments.

"Since this disease has gone all over, you cannot just focus on the lungs, where it started," said the master. "Instead, you have to focus on every channel of the body. You have to focus external Qi on all twelve meridian channels to increase the body's immune system so it can heal itself."

He also advised that I use my Qi energy "like radiation" to fight specific tumors like the one that was in the lung.

I went back to Shanghai and began Qi treatments the very next day. I administered external Qi over his entire body, emitting Qi from my fingertips, which were held approximately six inches away from each of the meridian points.

After I did this, the patient was much more relaxed. He

slept peacefully all afternoon, which was something his wife said he had not done for weeks. To me this meant that both his pain and his fear had subsided.

I continued the treatments.

After a couple of days, I had him start doing Qi Gong exercises. A few days later I combined the external and internal Qi treatments with herbs, including portions of cotyledon, which fights lung cancer. He took his medicine three times a day, did exercises twice a day, and had external Qi treatment from me twice a week. After eighteen months of steady improvement, he was considered cured by doctors at the hospital.

I was extremely excited by what had happened. I knew that this man had almost no chance of living for eighteen months, let along being cured of his disease. To me this was the best thing that could ever happen, and I was elated as I told Master Kwan about the final results.

"Don't think that this is going to happen every time you deal with a cancer patient," he said. "What happened here is great, but healing someone with cancer all over his body is extremely rare. Usually, the most you can do for him is increase the length of time that he is going to live and reduce his pain. What happened this time was the exception."

Still, it was the exception that aroused substantial curiosity. Some of the doctors thought the patient's cancer had been misdiagnosed and that he did not really have cancer to begin with. The ones who did the diagnosing insisted they had made no mistake. This man had been dying of cancer, they declared, and Qi Gong had healed him.

In the midst of this controversy, I was approached by two researchers from a nearby heart institute. They had research money already allotted and a flowering interest in Qi Gong. They wanted to know if I was willing to test my external Qi on patients who were possible candidates for coronary bypass surgery.

I would administer external Qi during a medical test known as angiography. In this test, radioactive dye is injected into the bloodstream so the amount of blood that flows through the heart can be accurately measured, both visually on a television screen and with sensitive instruments. The purpose of this test is to determine the blood flow to the heart by seeing how much the arteries are clogged.

The question these doctors were trying to answer was: Can external Qi improve blood flow in patients who may need bypass surgery? To answer that question, they would administer the dye test before and after I had emitted external Qi into the patients' chests. By doing this, they could clearly measure the effects of external Qi.

On the day of the test, I was taken to the angiography room. Technicians brought the first patient in and catheterized him, a process of stringing a tube into the large femoral artery in the thigh and up to the heart. It is through this tube that the dye that is to measure the pumping volume is delivered to the heart.

I stood over the patient while the technicians started the imaging camera that would film the heart in action. I could see it on a television screen, and then as the dye was injected into the bloodstream and passed through the chambers of the heart.

The doctors nodded to me from behind a window and I pointed my fingers at the patient's chest. He did not know what I was doing, nor do I think he cared. He was heavily sedated and was having trouble keeping his eyes open.

After I had emitted Qi for about thirty seconds, dye was released again. I could see the ghostlike image of the dye flow through the chambers of the heart. Film was taken and measurements were made. Then the patient's catheter was removed and another patient was brought in.

I emitted Qi into about six patients on that day. All the while I marveled at finally being able to bring this ancient healing art into the high-tech world of a cardiology lab.

Meanwhile, the researchers marveled at the results. In every patient, blood flow had increased and the heart rate slowed down during the Qi emission.

One of the doctors became very excited. "We have captured Qi on film," he said. "We have actually seen it affect human hearts."

This study had proven that *something* happened when Qi was emitted into a sick heart. Now the government was ready to see just what else could be done with this traditional medicine. After that, things began to happen very quickly. The government earmarked funds to study the effects of Qi on cancer.

In one of these studies, cancer cells were cultivated in a number of petri dishes. The dishes were then divided into two groups: those that were to be exposed to external Qi that I and other Qi Gong practitioners would emit, and those that would receive no emitted Qi. The point of this experiment was to see if emitted Qi had any effect upon living cancer cells.

The first time the experiment was done, the Qi practitioners emitted their Qi for five minutes into the individual cell cultures. A substantial number of cancer cells were killed in each of the cell cultures exposed to emitted Qi. Meanwhile, the cell cultures that were not exposed continued to thrive.

This experiment was repeated using ten minutes of emitted Qi on cell cultures, and then fifteen minutes. With each increased use of Qi, there was an increased number of cancer cells killed in the petri dishes.

That was proof that emitted Qi could kill cancer in petri dishes.

We then tried these experiments on animals with cancer. Dogs, rabbits, and rats were injected with cancer cells and then given time to let the cancer develop. A large number of animals developed cancer—well over one hundred. These animals were divided randomly into two groups: the ones that were to receive emitted Qi and those that were not. Once a day, the Qi practitioners would stand over the cages of the experimental group of animals and emit Qi. Even Master Kwan came down from the mountain to participate in this experiment. We did this for twenty to thirty minutes. Other than that, both animal groups were treated and fed the same.

We followed this procedure for two months, during which time many of the animals that did not receive external Qi died of their disease. To us, this meant that the survival time of the experimental group was longer than that of the control group. Survival time was not a part of the study, however. After two months, the animals were killed and dissected so the progress of their disease could be examined by a pathologist.

The results were astounding. Seventy-five percent of the animals that received emitted Qi had tumors much smaller than the ones that did not receive the Qi. The disease had also spread to a lesser degree in the experimental group than in the control.

This study has been duplicated several times since then with similar results. At the time, however, it caused quite a stir among cancer specialists. Always interested in treatments that will give them the edge against this seemingly unstoppable disease, cancer specialists became the greatest supporters of Qi Gong. They suggested that Qi Gong be used in conjunction with chemotherapy and radiation treatments to see if it could improve the effects of these treatments.

The Qi Gong masters, of course, already knew the answer. They had been using Qi Gong treatments on cancer patients for years. Many of these treatments had to be done in secret, since the medical doctors did not want their patients using any therapy other than their own. There were stories about cancer specialists stopping their treatments if they found out that an alternative form of treatment like Qi Gong was being used.

"For all these years these guys didn't want us," said Master Kwan. "Now that they have seen how good Qi Gong is, they want us to join them."

I could not argue with what he said. I had now been transferred to the tumor center of a large hospital in Shanghai. During the experiments, I had done especially well with tumors, and since tumors are so hard to deal with, I was immediately placed at a Qi Gong research center where I could do the most good.

Almost all of the patients there were being treated with Western methods, chemotherapy and radiation. I was brought in to add an extra dimension to cancer treatments, because the limits of Western cancer therapy are quite clear. Since chemotherapy and radiation are poisonous, too much of either will kill a patient.

Since Qi Gong is nonlethal, I could use it to push the attack even further. It was often the difference between survival and death, between more pain and less, and between more or less quality of life. Over the years I have treated more than five thousand cancer patients and I have no doubt through personal observations that Qi Gong made a positive difference in every one of my patients. I am firmly convinced that a combination of Western and Eastern medicine is the most effective means of treating cancer.

At the very least, Qi Gong and herbs can eliminate many of the side effects of chemotherapy, such as sores in the mouth and throat or diarrhea. I told my cancer patients then what I tell them now: "You may not have a choice about taking chemotherapy, but you do have a choice about suffering its side effects."

At the very most, I realized that Qi Gong might actually be the treatment that turns the illness around for a cancer patient. I do not say this to build up false hope, and I do not mean to imply that Qi Gong is a secret weapon that will win the battle over cancer every time. But at the same time I do want to say that it is an effective tool in fighting cancer, and may be the key to boosting the immune system, which is what fights cancer most effectively, anyway.

I say this because I have seen many miracle cures and remissions attributed to Qi Gong. In fact, my first official patient at the tumor center was one such case.

As had happened to an earlier patient, his cancer had started in his lung and moved throughout his body. By the time he was assigned to me, his cancer extended even into the bones of his legs and skull. Everything that could be done had already been done, including lung surgery, chemotherapy, and radiation.

The only thing left to do was Qi Gong, and frankly I had my doubts about how much effect that would have. After all, even Qi Gong has its limits. I remember reading the patient's file while his physician talked to me about the case.

"I am sorry that this has to be your first case," he said. "By my estimate he has about one month to live. Do what you can do. I don't think anyone will hold it against you if he doesn't make it."

I began treatment as I had been taught by Master Kwan. I administered external Qi twice a week for at least thirty minutes. My goal was to improve the functioning of his immune system while also treating specific cancer sites. To do this I worked on blocked meridians while also emitting Qi directly at certain tumors. Then I prescribed a very powerful herbal remedy and had him drink it three times per day.

Within a few weeks, just as this patient should have been dying, he was out of bed and performing Qi Gong exercises. I worked him very hard, doing many moving exercises that would strengthen his yang (or active) energy, and many meditation exercises to strengthen his yin (inactive) energy. These meditations are aimed at guiding energy through specific meridian channels. With meridians that are charged with Qi, the body will fight disease more readily.

When his doctor saw him exercising, he examined the patient thoroughly and pronounced him in a state of remission. He did not hesitate for one moment in crediting Qi Gong as being the therapy that tipped the scales in favor of healing.

Six months later medical tests showed that the cancer that had spread throughout his body had now diminished. The main tumor, which had started it all, had shrunk to about one-third its original size.

After one year, the cancer was completely gone.

The patient's physician was so pleased that he published the case study in a medical journal. Ten years later, in 1989, he presented the patient's case at the World Cancer Association Conference in Houston.

Since the events I have just related, there have been hundreds of studies conducted on the health effects of Qi Gong. To my knowledge, not one of these studies shows ill effects of Qi Gong on any patient, and virtually every study done on cancer and Qi Gong shows that it improves a cancer patient's status in many ways.

Thumbing through studies that are sitting on my desk right now, I can see that Qi Gong treatments can increase white blood cell counts, improve the functioning of the immune system, reduce pain, improve patient outlook, and increase life expectancy. Many studies show that Qi projection alone shrinks tumors and kills cancer cells in vitro. Combined with Western medicine, the effects of Qi treatment are increased.

Why is it that one treatment complements another so well? After years of using both approaches to treat patients, I think the answer is this: In traditional Chinese medicine, we consider cancer a local reflection of an overall imbalance in the body. So we fight disease by improving the immune system and increasing energy flow through the meridians. Western medicine, on the other hand, attacks the cancer itself with less regard to other parts of the body. Allopathic physicians will launch an attack on specific sites using approaches like chemotherapy or radiation. They may kill the cancer with this approach, but in the process they may damage organs, reduce the immune response, and deplete energy stores to critical levels, leaving the body vulnerable to further disease.

In my experience I have found that a combined approach to cancer is preferable. While Qi Gong builds the body's natural disease-fighting capacity, the Western medicine attacks the disease itself.

This is a somewhat simplified explanation, but one that helps us understand why patients who combine Eastern and Western therapies have greater odds in their battle against cancer.

6

The Mission

In the midst of this scientific interest in Qi Gong, word arrived that I was wanted by Master Kwan. A messenger came to the hospital with a note signed by the master that said simply, "Come to the mountain."

I was not at all surprised to receive such a communiqué. I had followed Master Kwan for eight years now and had come to expect the unexpected. I remembered the early days, when such a demand would have raised my blood pressure with anger and even would have caused me to curse the fact that I had ever gotten involved with someone so demanding as a Qi Gong master.

That attitude changed over the years as I realized that with every one of the master's demands there also came a learning experience. If I spent hours on the train to Canton, I would receive teaching from the master that would be well worth the inconvenience. If I worried about the patients I would not see at the hospital, I then found that I would see many more patients at the cave.

Rather than fight the course that my life had taken, I began to relax and flow with it. Master Kwan noticed this and one day said, "Rough water is not so rough when you swim with it. It is when you fight it that it becomes truly rough and takes all of your energy."

What he said put into words my changed attitude. I began to go with the flow of life, and when I did that, my mind cleared and I could see lessons in everything. For example, instead of asking why I was doing the Qi Gong exercises so often, I asked myself what it was I could learn by doing them so long. That made me direct my energy toward the positive aspects of my task and in turn gave me greater opportunity for knowledge.

As my view of life changed, so did my effect on patients. I found that I was able to guide the patients' attitude from negative to positive. If they looked at disease as a learning experience, then it was possible to make the disease process itself much less unpleasant. The lessons they could learn through illness involved everything from lifestyle changes to spiritual changes.

"It is important to relax as best you can during illness," I began to tell my patients. "When you are filled with stress and fear, then the cells of your body don't respond the way they are supposed to. Sometimes they become stagnant and don't respond at all. When that happens, you have real problems."

So when I received Master Kwan's request to come to the cave, I thought nothing of making immediate travel plans. After all, I had followed this man for eight years. Why leave the path now?

When I arrived at the cave, something was clearly afoot. Many of the apprentices came out to greet me as I walked up the path, but they were silent about why they were so happy.

The Mission

"What is going on?" I asked one of the apprentices.

"It is not for me to say," he replied. "But it is good news."

Soon we were joined by Master Kwan. I was quite nervous by now and was made even more so by the piercing gaze that I received from my master.

"It is your time to climb the ladder," he said. "I am making you a master tonight."

I was elated at the news. I had studied for years with little thought of becoming a master. I knew that, like other things in my life, it would come but only if I did not push for it. Suddenly, it was my time to become a master. I was both elated and overwhelmed by the responsibility, and I felt the sense of both burden and happiness at the same time.

"Do not worry," said Master Kwan, seeing the feelings in the look on my face. "You will still receive guidance from me. As a master, you still climb the ladder. You climb the ladder all of your life because you are always learning something new."

That night Master Kwan staged the ceremony that graduated me to the rank of master. I cannot tell you what the ceremony consists of, because it is one of the most secret ceremonies in the world and is known to only a few. I can repeat just the final few sentences of what Master Kwan said on the mountaintop that night, words that served as a kind of welcome to the world of mastery.

"When the heart is pure, it is in tune with the universe's energy and moves this limitless energy through yourself to help others," he said. "When you have reached this, you are in the way of Tao, the way of enlightenment. What I give to you as a teacher is but a starting point. Everything else you have to work for."

I became a Qi Gong master in 1979. Over the next several years I worked with thousands of cancer patients and eventually moved to the prestigious Shanghai Red Cross Hospital. I was a restless soul, "always on the path of learning," as Master Kwan put it. I would join him for interesting cases, no matter where the case might be. Sometimes we would catch an airplane and fly to a distant province to treat high government officials. One time, I was "requested" by the government to take care of a very old official who was sick. I was taken to his house in Beijing, where I was told by his assistants that I would have to live there in his house until I healed him. I had no choice. I was treated with all the respect given to dignitaries, and even given limited telephone privileges, but I was not allowed to leave.

Although I was told to consider this treatment an honor, I felt as though I were under virtual house arrest for three months before this man's problems improved.

Even though that kind of treatment by the government angered me, I loved the work I was doing and was pleased with the results we were having in our pioneering efforts to combine Eastern and Western medicine. I never thought of trying to leave the country.

One day I was called in to the main hospital by one of the head doctors. There in his office were a number of other doctors looking down at medical reports they held in their laps. In the midst of all these white coats was a frail, almost birdlike woman. She was wearing a hat and had the translucent skin and sallow look of someone who was exhausted by illness. Through remote diagnosis I could tell that her illness was breast cancer.

"This is Amy from Los Angeles in the United States," said the head doctor. "She has come here to see if we can help her."

Amy's story was a sad one. She was a medical doctor who had ignored a lump in her own breast almost two years earlier. By the time she went to a colleague to have it examined, the cancer had begun to spread to other parts of her body.

She immediately had a radical mastectomy and was started on chemotherapy. Still the cancer spread to her liver, lungs, kidneys, and bones until she had what is known as grade four cancer. Finally her physician said that doctors could not stop the disease and gave her approximately one month to live.

Amy decided not to give up.

She began to search for alternative therapies that could help with her cancer. She discovered the mountain of Qi Gong research that was coming out of China. She had read this research thoroughly and spoke very knowledgeably about it through an interpreter. Being trained under the Western medical system, she could not totally relate to the notion that our health and well-being had anything to do with "these things you Chinese call meridians."

Still, she said, she could not deny the results of the research. Especially impressive to her were studies showing emitted Qi killing cancer cells. By now many studies had been done in which tumors in animals were shrunk by Qi. Other studies done on humans showed improvement of those cancer patients who had Qi Gong therapy over those who did not. Not only did they live longer than the cancer patients who did not receive Qi Gong treatments, but they also experienced much less pain.

Many of these studies had their "miracle patients," ones who beat cancer using Qi Gong. In one case a woman with lung cancer that had metastasized began Qi Gong after radical surgery to remove the diseased lung. In subsequent checkups, doctors found the cancer had ceased to spread. In another case study a man with cancer of the esophagus began Qi Gong therapy as part of his treatment. A combination of chemotherapy and Qi Gong led to a complete disappearance of his cancer.

Amy hoped to become one of those miracle patients, although she was realistic in her assessment of her chances.

"I know my chances of recovery are slim," she said. "But I have to try."

I was assigned her case, which I considered a challenge as well as an opportunity. Although the popularity of Qi Gong as an effective treatment was spreading rapidly throughout the medical community in China, it had not yet gotten attention in the United States. If I could successfully treat an American physician with cancer, then surely she would return to her country and tell everyone what had happened. Such a healing would be like planting a seed in a distant land and having it turn into a grove of trees.

I began treatment immediately.

At first I performed emitted Qi treatments. I did this for more than thirty minutes, directing Qi at specific cancer sites. I also worked on her meridians, attempting to unblock those channels that were most affected by the disease. This, I explained to her, would give her greater overall health, which many cancer patients lack.

I prescribed a number of herbs as well. I will discuss them in more detail later, but in general terms these herbs were aimed at accomplishing three things:

- Increasing overall strength and supporting the body's good energy. This was accomplished by a number of herbs and other medicines, including rehmannia root, asparagus root, fleeceflower, and gelatin.
- Getting rid of elements that enhance the growth of the cancer. Some of the herbal remedies that do this are persica seed, salvia root, brassica seed, and minerals provided by oyster shell and pumice.
- Supporting the production of blood cells after radiation or chemotherapy. This is one example of Eastern medicine working in conjunction with Western medicine. Some of

the blood cell enhancers include licorice, asparagus root, and adenophora root.

To help open her body's energy meridians, I had her perform a number of Qi Gong exercises every day. These were exhausting at first, but I had her do them anyway.

"This is part of your fight," I told her. "These three things help each other in the fight against cancer."

Amy made great progress. After one month of treatment we had a party to celebrate the fact that she had outlived her physician's prognosis. The doctors and nurse on her ward all gathered in her room and toasted her and wished her long life. She was all smiles. By then she was looking much better. She had gained weight and much of her pain had diminished. The Qi Gong exercises had given her strength and skin tone, and I believe they enhanced the effects of all of the other aspects of treatment.

This is not to say that her life was wonderful, because it was not. People who are very sick have only one concern, and that is to get well. It is like a twenty-four-hour job for them, and it is a job that is not easy. She continued to take chemotherapy, and battled her loss of strength with Qi Gong exercises and meditations, which she practiced several times daily.

She improved gradually. After three months her blood composition had returned to nearly normal and she was recovering at a steady rate.

Then something happened that disrupted her healing.

I had noticed that Amy did not have contact with anyone back in the United States. In many ways she seemed to live in a shell. Although she was a pleasant person to be around, she never talked about her family. When I asked about them she would change the subject or simply say that she did not get along well with her parents. I thought this was wrong. She should try to come to an understanding with her parents. To fight with them now could only make her problems worse.

"Many diseases have emotional causes," I said. "If you let anger build up inside of you, it erupts in the form of disease."

She understood what I was saying, but still she never opened up about her family matters.

Then one day I came into Amy's room to find her crying. "What is wrong?" I asked.

"A horrible thing has happened in Los Angeles," she said, drying her eyes. "Since I have not contacted anyone in our family, they presumed I was dead. Our family lawyer filed papers saying that I died in China and now has plans to execute my will."

She found this out after telephoning her mother to tell her how much better she was doing. Not only had her mother told her about the mistake, but Amy felt that she did not sound especially happy to hear her voice.

I tried to put the events into perspective. Now that the truth was known, I said, surely the lawyer would undo what he had started. And besides, I added, whatever possessions Amy had were only material and certainly could not buy her the health she was now regaining.

I know that intellectually Amy had no problem understanding my argument. Everyone knows that ultimately they cannot buy good health. Still, Amy's material possessions were very important to her. She was raised in a family in which wealth played a prominent role, and asking her to ignore her possessions would be like asking her to change identities.

"I have to go back home and settle this," she insisted. "What they did is just wrong."

For days I argued with Amy, but to no avail. I told her that the stress of dealing with her family might bring her cancer out of remission. "You are doing so well, why risk it?"

When I realized that, to Amy, it was worth the risk, I mixed up a large batch of herbs for her trip and wrote out some prescriptions that she could have filled at any one of the many Chinese pharmacies in Los Angeles. I gave her a number of Qi Gong exercises to do each day and suggested that she take meditation breaks from any situation that might seem stressful. If she took such breaks, I reasoned, it might keep the stress from snowballing into bigger problems.

"Most of all, take care of yourself," I said. "Come back in good shape."

She did come back, but not in good shape. Six weeks later Amy returned looking every bit as ill as when she arrived the first time. Medical tests showed that her cancer had returned with a vengeance and appeared to be spreading again. Her family situation had improved, but it had still taken its toll on her. She had been involved in angry fights with her lawyer about his actions and had also fought considerably with her father. I got the idea that Amy came from a family whose competitiveness knew no bounds. They competed not only with people outside of their family, but with each other as well. Such competition may have served Amy well at some points in her life, but now she needed compassion.

After a few days of rest, we started the treatments all over again. Even though she had deteriorated, Amy responded to treatment very well. She admitted that she had spent little time doing the Qi Gong exercises I had asked her to do in the United States. As far as the meditations went, she did none of that.

"I did take the herbs," she said in defense of herself. "But I guess that was not enough."

Again we were able to balance Amy's physical state. She

became much stronger as we continued the treatments that we had done the first time she came to Shanghai.

And so it went for many more months. Amy was feeling so much better after her first few weeks that she moved into a hotel room and came to the hospital as an outpatient. I saw her at least twice a week. I would administer my Qi treatments and give her new exercises if she needed them.

Although Amy improved physically, I could not say the same for her mental state. This time she continued to keep in touch with her family, but she fought a lot with her parents on the telephone. I did not know the specifics of what was going on, only that it was extremely upsetting to Amy.

At the end of one of her appointments, Amy announced that she was leaving China and returning to the United States. She felt that the most important thing in her life was her business interests, mainly the large amount of real estate she and her family owned.

"Now that I am better, I need to go back home and take care of my life," she said.

What could I say? I told her that the trip might cause more mental stress than she was already experiencing. I tried to gently coax her into staying in Shanghai for a few more months. But in the end I was ineffective. All I could do was write her herbal prescriptions, give her specific diet plans, and encourage her to do her Qi Gong exercises every day.

I felt helpless to control her and reluctant to tell her the truth, which was simply this: The only business she should focus on was the business of her own personal health. At home, she would experience a great deal of stress through her difficult relationship with her parents and siblings. The spoken word can be bad medicine just as it can be good. Environment can hurt or heal a patient just as surely as strong medication.

I did not feel well the day she left. I felt as though I would never see her again.

Several months later I received a telephone call from David Chang, the vice consulate for the United States in Shanghai. He told me the sad news that Amy had died in Los Angeles.

"You must have been very close to her," he said.

"She was a patient," I said.

"She must have thought very highly of you," he said. "She has made you the sole beneficiary of her estate. I don't know the particulars, but I think you are a very rich man."

I was stunned. On the one hand I had always wanted to see the United States, which was rich and free beyond my wildest imaginings. If I went there, this would be a chance to see another part of the world and exchange ideas on the healing arts. On the other hand, it was not the traditional Chinese way to take someone's fortune. If there is still family living, then that is where the fortune should stay, no matter how bad the relationship between them might be. To break up a family fortune would bring bad luck to all concerned.

The vice consulate made plans for me to go to Los Angeles immediately. Amy's family had a considerable amount of political clout, he said, and they insisted upon getting this matter cleared up immediately. Within a few weeks, I had a passport and travel visa for the United States. I planned to be there only a short period of time, but I wanted to see Master Kwan before I left. Luckily, he was coming to Shanghai and I was able to see him.

He came to my mother's house and we talked about the strange events leading up to my upcoming trip to America. At one point I mentioned that I would try to bring back some merchandise for him that was difficult to get in mainland China. He just shrugged when I said this and looked at me with a sly grin.

"Maybe you will not come back at all," he said. "Maybe you will find a void there that only you can fill."

"What do you mean?" I asked. "What kind of void?"

"If you see it you will know what I mean," he said. He then said some things that seemed very cryptic to me at the time and that I will mention later. Now they make perfect sense, but when he said them, I felt as though he was talking to someone else and not me.

A few days later I left Shanghai.

I had friends in the United States who met me at the airport. These were people I knew while growing up in Shanghai. They had been in America for some time and had very different ideas about what I should do with the fortune Amy had left me.

"You would be crazy to turn it down," one of my friends said. "Forget tradition and live here as a wealthy man."

I understood what he was saying. I met with Amy's lawyers once, and they told me that her estate consisted of a great deal of property in Newport Beach. Then I listened as they threatened to take me to court and challenge Amy's right to leave her wealth to me. My lawyer, who was recommended by my friend, told them that they had no grounds on which to challenge the will. Then I told them I did not want to listen anymore. I told them I would make my decision in two weeks.

Of course I had already made my decision: I would not accept the fortune no matter what. But I did not want to tell them my decision just yet. I wanted to stay in the United States as long as possible. I was intrigued by the culture and attracted by the fact that there was a great interest in Qi

Gong. Already word had spread throughout the Chinese community that a Qi Gong master was in town, and people were coming to the house where I was staying for treatments. One day I came home to find a number of people sitting on the front step. The friend I was staying with was perplexed by the sudden influx of patients. "I didn't know you would turn my house into a hospital," he said. Even though he said it with good humor, there was real concern in his eyes. This is not what he thought would happen when he took me in as a houseguest.

Two weeks later I went back to the law firm that represented Amy's family. I went with a few friends of mine from the Chinese community. One of them served as interpreter and the others just wanted to witness this spectacle. They still could not believe that I was going to renounce this windfall from a grateful patient and they wanted to see firsthand what happened.

After we had sat in the waiting room for an uncomfortable period of time, a very cool secretary ushered us into a beautifully appointed conference room. Surrounding the table were a number of lawyers in suits that were pressed smooth and looked like armor. Amy's sister was there, too. She was Amy's business partner and was spearheading this legal effort to keep Amy's estate within the family. They all looked like nervous warriors and they became more tense when I smiled. How else could they have been? Much of their family empire was on the line and that would be enough to make anyone emit negative Qi.

I got right to the point.

"I appreciate Amy's feelings when she left me her estate," I said through an interpreter. "As you can see from what she wrote in her will, she felt abandoned by her family and friends and struggled with that rejection until the end of her life. I, in turn, gave her hope and support and made her physically and emotionally healthier, which is what she truly needed. But even though I understand why she left me her estate, I cannot accept it. I am a Taoist, and it would not be my way to break up a family's fortune."

There was shock all around the table. I think they were expecting a great battle and were not prepared for the realization that it would not occur even though that was reason for happiness.

A release was written, I signed it, and then the burden of Amy's estate was lifted from my shoulders. Amy's holdings were quite extensive and included more than 150 apartments in Newport Beach. Still I do not regret refusing her generous offer. To have accepted it would have gone against my beliefs.

One afternoon I thought back to my last conversation with Master Kwan and suddenly realized what he was talking about when he mentioned the void that only I could fill. That void was a lack of Qi Gong masters, one that I could begin to fill by staying in America.

During this time I also met a beautiful Chinese woman named Alice. I was attending a banquet one night at a huge Chinese restaurant and happened to be seated at a big round table with a number of people, including Alice and her two children. I was talking about Qi Gong with a number of people at the table when Alice began to say that she did not believe in remote diagnosis. I could understand her skepticism. Since she had been raised in the United States, she had never seen it done.

"I will show you," I said. Immediately I did a remote diagnosis of her children, both of whom had been to the doctor recently for specific complaints. The accuracy of the diagnosis silenced Alice and brought several of the people at the table to me as patients the very next week. As you say in this country, "Seeing is believing." I became busier than ever.

A few weeks later, Alice came to me as a patient. She had broken her ankle while playing tennis and was now being told by her physician that surgery would be necessary to repair the break. She did not want to have surgery and wondered if there was anything I could do to help her avoid it.

I prepared an herbal poultice and applied it to her ankle. I told her to leave it on for three days and that would take care of the problem. After two days the area underneath the poultice began to itch so much that she removed it. After that she did not need the surgery, but the ankle still bothers her on rainy days. I know that is only because she took the poultice off a day early.

After that, Alice became one of my students and began to study Qi Gong. Less than one year later we were married.

My practice has expanded in ways that I never thought possible. My patients include doctors, lawyers, electrical engineers, athletes, college students, and Hollywood stars. These are all very different types of people, but still they are bound together by the common need for good health.

I do the best I can to take care of that need.

Sometimes, though, I am lonely for my homeland. I miss the culture of my birth and its rich sense of history. I miss my mother and the discussions about health and science that were ongoing in our home. I look back at those discussions with a great fondness and realize that they are my very foundation and the reason that my curiosity about the mystery of life has never stopped growing. Those discussions were like an endless stage play, one that I could join at any point. That play is still onstage at my mother's home. At times I feel sad knowing that I will never be a part of it again.

To keep from longing for the old days, I think about the future and I become very excited. There is much to do in my new home. I have been here since 1990 and have already trained hundreds of students in the art of Qi Gong. I have also treated thousands of patients with all kinds of diseases— from cancers and AIDS, to strokes, heart disease, and daily stress.

My life is rich and full, but still I am never complacent, because there is always more to explore. The message of Master Kwan is imprinted in my mind.

"The path to Tao has just begun for you," he told me that last time I saw him in Shanghai. "Do not think that you have learned everything already, because there is always someone more able than you from whom you can learn. No one is perfect, which is why you must go out and travel to learn as much as you can. I am giving you three missions that you must accomplish:

"First, you must do good and help those in need.

"Second, you must gather the Qi of different areas so you can understand the world and become a better master. All things have Qi energy that can take on a physical form when you relax and absorb the energy of the universe. Qi creates all things and all things revert back to Qi.

"Finally, you must learn and exchange what you have learned, and in doing so make friends as you go."

I have stayed on the path set by my master. I will stay on it until I reach my end.

PART II

Studies in Healing

7

The Practice of Qi Gong

The principle of Yin and Yang is the basic principle of the entire universe. It is the root and source of life and death; and it is also found within the temples of the gods.
—THE YELLOW EMPEROR'S CLASSIC
OF INTERNAL MEDICINE

Even though *The Yellow Emperor's Classic of Internal Medicine* is widely considered the beginning of Chinese medicine, it is in no way the final word. Written as a conversation between the emperor and his physicians, this work represents medical knowledge as it was known to the ancients. But much of it was written nearly four thousand years ago. And just as allopathic medicine has evolved since the times of Hippocrates, so has Chinese medicine.

Trial and error have changed the nature of Qi Gong and other forms of traditional Chinese medicine and continue to do so even now. As with Western medicine, evolution never stops and perfection is never attained. A good physician is always looking for a better and more effective way to heal his patients. It is the ever-changing quality of medicine and the differences between patients that make the practice of being a physician an art as well as a science.

When I look at the Qi Gong exercises that the ancient masters used, I can see that they provided the foundation for the exercises the masters of today prescribe. We have taken the essence of these ancient exercises and improved upon them.

The same is true of the herbal formulas. The ancients discovered the basic properties of many plants, but it took thousands of years of trial and error to discover how these plants could be combined into the highly effective herbal remedies we now use.

Such evolution of knowledge will continue for as long as humans exist.

To illustrate the Qi Gong approach to medicine, I have selected several case studies that show the course of treatment I have taken with illnesses, ranging from chronic problems like headaches and allergies to such life-threatening diseases as AIDS and hypertension.

As you will see, I combine Qi, herbs, and food to attack disease on all fronts and to balance the body's yin and yang. The goal of Qi Gong—and all forms of traditional Chinese medicine, for that matter—is to return a patient to a state of "radiant health." This means simply that a person has become so healthy that he or she is beyond danger of falling further victim to illness.

Achieving radiant health involves the intervention of herbs, food, and even the external Qi that I use to boost a patient's own Qi. But my treatment also relies on the patient himself for much of the healing that takes place. As I told one patient: "In Qi Gong, the patient is considered the soldier

who fights his illness. By the same analogy, the d
sidered the commander. I will give you
weapons and your marching orders, but you have
of the fighting."

By telling patients this I am saying that they must comply
with all of my medical orders. Of course, they must do the
exercises and take the herbs, and they must do so faithfully
and ignore the temptations not to "take their medicine."
American medical studies show that most patients do not
follow their doctor's orders to the letter, yet they blame the
doctor if their illness is not cured.

Achieving radiant health requires compliance. But it also
requires something more of the patient. I ask that my patients
look for signs of improvement and build upon them. In part
this is a way of encouraging positive thinking, which has a
very large role in healing. But it is also a way of building on
your strengths.

"When you are sick, it is easy to think about how bad you
feel and not pay attention to the times you feel good," I tell
my patients. "Analyze carefully the times you feel good. They
are bright spots in illness but they sometimes hold the key to
making you feel even better."

What follows is a case study of one of my most compliant patients. I have presented it in detail, so you can see
specifically how both the patient and I approach a disease
successfully.

In this case I have chosen a patient who had prostate cancer. I consider all forms of healing a miracle. But the most
miraculous for me has been those times when Qi Gong has
slowed and even stopped cancer.

A man I will call Raymond arrived at my clinic dizzy
with fear. His doctor had just given him the results of a test
that told him he had advanced prostate cancer. The doctor

wanted to perform surgery to remove the gland. This procedure, known as radical prostatectomy, would likely leave him
incontinent and rob him of his sexual abilities. The doctor
said he had little choice, however. Without effective treatment, the cancer would likely spread throughout his body
and end his life. Raymond did not want either of these
events to happen. He was clearly in a corner with few places
to turn.

Raymond had heard of me through friends and decided
to try traditional Chinese medicine before having surgery.
He was very nervous as he sat across from me in my examining room. He showed me the results of the medical tests his
doctor had conducted. I could see from one in particular, the
prostate specific antigen test (PSA), that there was certainly
cancer in his prostate.

In addition to these medical tests, I used my Qi Gong
powers to scan him for other problems besides the cancer.
Beginning with his head and working down, I could see the
pattern of energy as it circulated throughout his meridians.
In Chinese medicine, energy circulates within the human
body through twelve meridians, or channels. An ancient
medical text explains this concept in poetic terms: "Heaven
is covered with the constellations, earth with waterways, man
with channels."

To a trained Qi Gong master, the energy surrounding a
person has a distinct appearance, almost like heat waves ris-
ing off hot pavement. Others have described Qi as looking
like a vapor or breath.

In Raymond, I could see the flow of good energy while
at the same time seeing where bad energy was concentrated.
I could also see where energy was blocked and not flowing
in his body.

Raymond had many problems he had not told me about.
Maybe he did not think they mattered, but I did. In Qi

Gong, the body is considered as a whole, with one part affecting others like a great spider web. I could see allergies in the redness of his eyes. Scanning lower, I could see bad energy coming from vertebrae in his neck as well as bad energy coming from vertebrae in the lower back that radiated pain throughout his hipbone. It was clear to me that both of these were caused by some kind of traumatic injury. I could also see that his bladder was dysfunctional, causing frequent and painful urination.

As I saw these areas of concern in Raymond, I made marks on a diagnostic sheet. On this sheet is the front and back outline of a man. I keep it in patients' files to serve as a visual reminder of what their problem areas are when they first come in, and how they change over intervening visits.

This technique of diagnosing a patient by scanning is puzzling for most Western patients. Some even think that I am reading their minds instead of their bodies. I can understand why it seems like extrasensory perception, but it really is not that at all. This diagnostic ability requires only that I know what I am looking for in the way of Qi channels. "You can do it yourself," I tell my apprentices. "All you have to do is study with a master for eight years."

"The energy fields that surround us can be visible to everyone," Master Kwan told me. "I am just here to show you how to discover them."

Still, this form of diagnosis gets patients' attention when they first experience it. Raymond was shocked that I could perceive other physical problems besides his prostate cancer. He looked at the marks on the diagnostic sheet and was surprised. "How do you know all of this?" he asked. Then he spoke with new enthusiasm. "Let's begin," he said.

First I had some explaining to do. Qi Gong treatments differ from other forms of treatment, I said. In Western medicine, disease is attacked with medications and surgical procedures while the underlying cause is often ignored. In Chinese medicine, it is believed that the symptoms of an illness can manifest themselves in an area that is very far from the root cause. If that cause is not discovered and treated, the symptoms will only return.

To give an example familiar to Western medicine, it is entirely possible to have a heart bypass operation without being counseled on the lifestyle factors that caused the artery blockage in the first place. A heart patient who does not know that proper diet and exercise can keep him off the operating table will most likely find himself in surgery again.

In Chinese medicine we believe that disease is just a local reflection of overall problems. In general terms, good health depends on the proper balance of yin and yang energies. Yin is seen as female, as well as dark and cold. Yang is male, light and hot. These two opposite energies exist in every living thing. One must strive for harmony of these energies to prevent or heal an illness.

Since traditional Chinese medicine is based on natural healing, the five elements of nature are frequently referred to by Chinese doctors. This springs from the theory that all phenomena in the universe relate to interaction between the five elements: wood, fire, earth, metal, and water. Since Chinese physicians see the human body as a smaller representation of the greater universe, we use the elements of nature as a metaphor to categorize parts of the body by the elements they most resemble. The following list shows the five elements and their corresponding organs:

Wood: Liver, gallbladder
Fire: Heart, small intestines
Earth: Spleen, stomach
Metal: Lung, large intestines
Water: Kidney, bladder

These elements interact in the corresponding organs of the body as they do in nature. For instance, fire burns wood, which becomes charcoal and returns to the earth. In the human body, the small intestines (fire) burn food that the liver (wood) has helped to digest.

These elements can also work against each other. In nature, metal can chop wood and water can extinguish fire. In the human body, the kidney (water) can malfunction in a disease known as high blood pressure and damage the heart (fire).

It is through these metaphors of nature that Chinese doctors explain the complex interactions that take place in the human being.

In diagnosing diseases, different types of energy are given different names known as the six evils: heat, cold, wind, dampness, dryness, and fire. There are internal conditions that are defined through the use of these diagnostic terms. For instance, actual dampness can cause joint pain in some people and would be considered an external evil that caused the disease. However, a diet consisting of too much junk food and caffeine would inhibit functioning of the organs, thus causing what we call internal dampness.

These evils are referred to throughout the case studies in this section. It is important to note that although these six states are called "evils," they are evil only if they occur out of season, or when or where they are not supposed to. As stated in *The Yellow Emperor's Classic of Internal Medicine,* "Where evil energy gathers, weakness occurs. . . . When pure energy flourishes, evil energy flees."

Just as imbalance between people and environment can cause illness, illness can be extinguished with a restoration of balance. This concept is summed up nicely in *The Commentary of Zuo,* a medical text written in 540 B.C.:

The six influences are yin, yang, the wind, dampness, darkness, and light. . . . An excess of yin causes chills; an excess of yang causes fever; an excess of wind causes ailments of the limbs; an excess of rain causes ailments of the stomach; an excess of darkness affects the mind; an excess of light affects the feelings.

For the most part, this balance is attained through the healing and mastery of your Qi. Such mastery is accomplished through Qi Gong exercises, changes in diet, and herbal medications. Herbs are the very backbone of any Chinese medical therapy. Herbal remedies have been in use for almost four thousand years in China. This has resulted in a trial-and-error system that has led to the most effective herbal remedies known to humankind.

A combination approach has always been considered necessary in Chinese medicine. So has the need to treat a disease early, before the symptoms become too extreme. This preventive approach to illness is emphasized as far back as the fifth century, when the physician Sun Simiao said, "Superior treatment consists of dealing with an illness before it appears; mediocre treatment consists of curing an illness on the point of revealing itself; inferior treatment consists of curing the illness once it has manifested itself."

This, of course, is a warning to both physician and patient.

Although Chinese medicine uses different terms and philosophies than its Western counterpart, its goal is essentially the same: to rid the body of illness and disease. It is in the approach to this common goal that the two systems show their differences.

In Western medicine, the patient is often passive and merely receives treatment. In Chinese medicine, the patient must be actively involved in his healing. We believe that if the patient will not participate in the fight against his disease, then the illness will likely take whatever course it wishes. It is that simple.

Raymond was glad to hear that I was a cancer specialist at the Shanghai Red Cross Hospital in China. As a practitioner at that large hospital, I was able to weave the two systems together, using the best of the East and the West to fight this disease. I treated hundreds of people with cancer of varying severity. In doing that I realized that traditional Chinese medicine and the treatments of the West join forces very well in the fight against disease.

"Imbalances in five main areas will cause cancer," I told Raymond. "Environmental, physical, chemical, biological, and psychological. To prevent a disease like cancer, one must watch his diet, maintain emotional stability, avoid pollution, and increase physical fitness. This will result in a high level of immune strength, which will get rid of the bad energy."

It is the mention of "good" and "bad" energy that usually makes Western doctors flinch. They are accustomed to thinking in terms of tissue and blood, and not the energy that permeates it. In Qi Gong it is the other way around. We look at this energy as the source of both health and illness.

In Qi Gong we believe that we are constantly being charged with energy. This energy comes from the earth and the sky, our workplace and home, even other people. It also comes from the things we eat, our activities, and even our psychological state. The combination of yin (passive) and yang (active) energy is Qi. The practice and study of Qi is Qi Gong.

I explained to Raymond that in Qi Gong, we try to balance the two energies, yin and yang, because balance is required in all aspects of life. Extremities in anything tend to cause problems.

Just as too much fatty food makes a person overweight, it

also gives him bad energy or blocks the flow of his energy entirely. People who work too hard also find themselves feeling angry and stressed, facing energy imbalances and blockages.

In Western medicine, prostate cancer is considered a hazard of aging. It is most common in men over the age of sixty and its cause is unknown. In Chinese medicine, we believe that prostate cancer is caused by blockages of the Sanjiao, kidney, and bladder meridians, which lead to abnormal urination as well as problems like prostate cancer.

To help Raymond overcome this energy blockage, I used Qi projection to open his meridians and improve his energy and blood circulation. This involves directing Qi from the universe through myself and into the affected area. If you have not seen this done, it looks quite bizarre. It involves the Qi Gong master pointing his finger at the areas that need energy in much the same way that you might point your fingers at someone if you were pretending to hold a gun. The difference here is that energy, not bullets, comes out of the Qi Gong master's fingers.

Patients of mine frequently feel heat or tingling inside their bodies while I am emitting Qi. Sometimes areas of their bodies quiver as I direct energy into them. This occurs even when I am standing behind a patient and they cannot see where it is that I am directing energy.

I have seen masters use external Qi to push plates across counters and to move tree branches on windless days. However, the most convincing demonstration of Qi to a Western audience might be the one that took place for a group of Harvard doctors in Beijing. They reported seeing a Qi Gong master at a cancer institute light a light bulb by holding it in his hands.

His superiors became angry at him for conducting such a demonstration. Such a use of Qi, they probably felt, was like having a doctor bring an X-ray machine to a party. Qi projection is not a parlor trick. It is a serious tool for healing.

With Raymond, I used this serious tool in three ways:

- To remove the bad energy.
- To force the bad energy out of the meridian exit points.
- To introduce good energy from the universe back into the meridians.

External Qi administered by a Qi Gong master functions as a sort of booster to the Qi Gong exercises. Once people learn the Qi Gong exercises, they do not need to have external Qi from a master. In most cases, external Qi is administered only to give them a head start on what the exercises will accomplish. This is generally true, although the greater the illness, the greater the need for external Qi, since sick people are not able to generate enough Qi on their own and often need help.

"I will give you the knowledge necessary to understand Qi Gong," I tell many of my patients and students. "But you must practice on your own to keep your meridians open."

After administering external Qi to Raymond, I outlined the specific methods of treatment I would use to bring his body back into balance:

The practice of specific exercises to get rid of the bad energy. Nearly everyone I treat receives a prescription for exercise. These exercises are very specific to a person' physical needs and are always aimed at opening the meridians. When Qi flows through the meridians, it ultimately enters every cell in the body. Without a steady flow of Qi, our bodies do not receive full nourishment. Each organ has its own meridian, and there is a meridian that affects each part of the body.

These meridians are much like rivers. When they are flowing well, then everything is fine. When they become obstructed through such factors as stress, poor diet, or bad environment, then the symptoms of pain and illness begin to occur. A rash, for instance, can be an early warning signal that a meridian is blocked. So can headaches, stomachaches, and the like.

The purpose of the exercises I prescribed to Raymond were to use movement in conjunction with the proper directing of the mind, body, and breath to unclog specific meridians and eliminate bad energy.

For this I had Raymond perform the Golden Eight Exercises described in the next chapter. Then I gave him three extra exercises aimed at directing good energy and improving blood circulation in his reproductive system.

Raymond took his role as a cancer fighter seriously. He performed these exercises two hours daily for three months. He was a diligent soldier, battling for his own health.

The use of specific foods and herbs to improve the body's balance. "Magical plants" have been the subject of legend in China for hundreds of years.

It was not until 1949, however, that the government started scientific research on the more than one thousand plants commonly used as medicine in China. It was then that they began to discover that the "myth" of herbal medicine translated into good science. Many of the plants they researched turned out to contain compounds present in allopathic medicine. A plant, *Scopola tangutica*, used since the second century, for instance, was found to be effective because it contained scopolamine, a commonly used analgesic. Another example is the herb Hwan Lian, which the Chinese use to treat earaches and intestinal disorders. An extract of this herb is used in the allopathic community to treat diarrhea, coughing, and ear infections. And then there is the herb Ma Huang, which has been used for thousands of years in China as part of anti-asthmatic formulas. It contains ephedrine, which is used in Western drugs for the same purpose. It is estimated that twenty-five percent of all prescription drugs in the United States originated from plants.

I am the first to admit that there are many ingredients that work in ways we do not understand. In defense of traditional Chinese medicine, however, I must point out that there are many Western drugs that work in unknown ways as well, including some of the actions of common drugs like aspirin. The point is that these herbal remedies work, and work quite well.

I do not recommend taking herbal remedies without discussing them first with your primary care physician. As with Western medicine, the first rule of the Chinese herbalist is to "do no harm." Before taking any of the herbal formulas in this book, make certain to discuss them with your doctor. And if you feel as though you are having an adverse reaction to the herbal formula, stop taking it immediately.

Even though herbs are natural and are usually more gentle than synthetic drugs, they are still a potent form of medication. Give them the respect that any powerful medication deserves.

The herbal remedies I prescribed for Raymond (presented in detail in the prostate cancer case study in Chapter 12) had five objectives:

- Nourish kidney energy and make the spleen healthy.
- Make urination easy and pain-free.
- Increase overall vitality and the spleen's yang energy.
- Balance the energy between the stomach and spleen.
- Rid the body of infection.

I also changed Raymond's eating habits. By eating properly, all of Raymond's energy could be directed toward fighting illness instead of digesting food, which is where much of our energy is expended on a daily basis. As part of his treatment package, I had him follow these strict guidelines for eating:

- Eat lots of vegetables, raw or cooked without oil.
- Eat whole grains with every meal.
- Eat lots of fruit.
- Do not eat rich desserts.
- Avoid foods with additives or preservatives.
- Drink pure water instead of soft drinks.
- Use sesame oil in place of butter or margarine.
- Steam, poach, broil, bake, or stir-fry with water, instead of using oil.
- Eat little meat.
- Snack frequently on vegetables.

As with all aspects of Chinese medicine, such dietary guidelines have strong links to the past. Even Confucius espoused dietary guidelines not too different from the ones I prescribed. "Be moderate in eating and drinking," the philosopher wrote. "Even if meat were abundant, one must not eat more meat than rice. Even with plenty still on the table, one must never eat more than is proper."

The specific healing regimen I prescribed for Raymond was the classic approach to illness taken by traditional Chinese medicine. It is covered in detail in the chapter on cancer.

I saw Raymond frequently after that first treatment session. Like a good patient, he followed my instructions explicitly. He tried not to fear his cancer. Instead he focused his attention on getting well and never strayed from my medical orders.

As the months passed I could see Raymond improving. He looked healthier and acted it, too. I am not saying that he had no fear. He was frightened of cancer and what it would mean if it progressed. Still, he was glad to be trying an approach to his disease that would not damage him for the rest of his life.

Three months after we began therapy, it was observed by Raymond's friends that he had regained his vitality as well as his appetite for both food and life. He reported that he was able to sleep well and, most important, was able to urinate without pain.

In my remote diagnosis of him, I could see very few traces of cancer remaining in his system. He seemed to be back to normal. At this point I told Raymond to go to his doctor for the blood test that would tell the truth about my Qi Gong treatments.

Even though I have waited many times for blood tests like this one, I still get nervous. All physicians get close to their patients, but Qi Gong masters get closer than most. I remember the words of my master: "Qi Gong is healing through the heart. Look beyond the wealth, fame, fortune, power, social placement, prior disgrace, hardship, and sense of gain or loss when treating. You have only compassion, love, and generosity when curing a patient. Only think about alleviating his pain." We work in harmony with our patients to help them through a disease. Because of this closeness, we are elated in their healing, and we feel their pain.

With Raymond there was elation. The blood tests administered by his Western physician showed an absence of the blood protein that meant cancer was present. Qi Gong had made another person well.

★ ★ ★

The case studies in the chapters that follow represent only a tiny glimpse inside the medical treasure chest that is Qi Gong. They illustrate my approach to a variety of illnesses. Each of these case studies includes Qi Gong exercises as well as the herbal remedies I used in the individual cases.

I am aware of the difficulties involved in finding herbal remedies in a nonherbal society like the United States. If you live in a major city that has a Chinatown district, chances are good that it will have an herbal pharmacy. If that is the case, bring this book to the pharmacist and show him the formula you want.

If you prefer to order these formulas through the mail, I have included in the Resources appendix three herbal suppliers who are familiar with the herbal formulas in this book. Feel free to contact them for a price list and a complete catalogue of their products.

Also included are recipes that the Chinese call "food cures." The Chinese have always been great believers in the healing properties of foods: Thousands of years ago, Chinese medical texts urged doctors to use medicine as a last resort "only when food fails."

As with herbs, foods are prescribed according to their qualities of "hotness" and "coolness" and their affinity for specific organ systems. Unlike Western food cures, which tend to be aimed at lowering fat and cholesterol intake, Chinese food cures promote the proper functioning of organs.

In China there are even restaurants where an herbalist tells you what to eat for an ailment. In some of these restaurants you could end up with a bowlful of chicken soup with ginseng for the flu, black ants on hash-brown potatoes or a stir-fried scorpion on toast for arthritis. Admittedly, Chinese tastes can be peculiar by Western standards. We, too, believe that "an apple a day keeps the doctor away." But eating ants or sometimes even turtle meat can do the same thing.

In this book, we have kept Western sensibilities in mind and have not included the more exotic medicinal recipes. Most of the recipes included are quite tasty, while others taste like, well, medicine. I tried to present a balance so you would know both the yin and yang of the healing foods of China.

Of course, not all people who study Qi Gong do so because they are ill. I have many patients who come because they are well and want to stay that way. These are my wellness patients, people who are using Qi Gong to stay youthful, supple, and strong.

I explain wellness this way: The human body is like a tree, with our feet and legs being the foundation of our well-being much like the roots of a tree are the foundation of its existence. The importance of a strong foundation in the feet and legs can be seen in both aging and illness, where the feet and legs are usually the first things to become weak. As we Chinese say, "We slowly die from our feet up."

My wellness patients know this and practice the Golden Eight Exercises that constitute the next chapter. These are exercises that emphasize the legs and feet, where all of the main meridians and channels either begin or end.

Because of their ability to strengthen and balance the entire body, you will notice that I recommend these eight exercises to the patients in all of the case studies.

Finally, I suggest that you have your doctor or health practitioner take a look at the treatments outlined here to make sure they are compatible with his or her goals. Qi Gong can be used in conjunction with most treatments administered by Western doctors, and I always have my patients talk to their physician in detail about what I have prescribed. In doing this I am making sure that the patient is getting the best care that the East and West have to offer.

8

The Golden Eight Exercises

*If man's vitality and energy do not propel his own will, his
disease cannot be cured.*
— THE YELLOW EMPEROR'S CLASSIC
OF INTERNAL MEDICINE

The Golden Eight Qi Gong Exercises have been the subject
of a number of medical studies around the world and have
been shown to be an excellent means of healing and health
maintenance. Each exercise is targeted at improving the
function of specific organs and eliminating illnesses. The
Golden Eight Exercises represent the primary internal exercises that balance yin and yang, and I recommend them to
many of my patients as a way to unblock the twelve meridian channels of the body. By unblocking these meridians,
many diseases can be prevented or treated.

A number of studies have examined the effects of these
(or similar) exercises on general health, and the exercises have
been found to have positive effects on everything from heart

function to aging. For the most part, these studies compared people who performed Qi Gong exercise routines at least three times per week, similar to the Golden Eight Exercises, with people who do other forms of exercise, like walking or running, or perhaps those who have no regular exercise routine. These studies examine the health of people before and after doing regular Qi Gong exercise. Some of them involved studying thousands of people, while others involved as few as twenty. All of them have shown that Qi Gong is extremely beneficial to overall health. Following is my summary of what these studies have found.

Cardiovascular effects. Regular practice of Qi Gong results in increased blood supply to the heart as well as stronger contractions of the heart muscle and a slower, more efficient heart rate. This increased blood supply improves the overall health of all of the body's organs. The improved heart function lowers the chances of hypertension and arteriosclerosis.

Respiratory effects. Qi Gong exercises increase the elasticity of lung tissue and improve the efficiency of the lungs themselves, allowing them to extract more oxygen from the air they breathe.

Effect on bones and muscles. Qi Gong exercises increase both muscle and bone strength as well as overall flexibility. In one study, the spines of twenty people who did Qi Gong exercises were compared with the spines of twenty who did not. The Qi Gong group had better posture than the non–Qi Gong group. They also had half the amount of bone loss and many times the spinal flexibility as a result of performing these exercises.

Effects on the central nervous system. There is a strong mind/body component to Qi Gong exercises, most likely due to the high degree of concentration required to do the exercises. Studies have shown that these exercises stimulate the cerebral cortex of the brain, causing, as one researcher put it, "excitation in certain parts and protective inhibitions in others." It is my belief that these exercises focus attention so deeply on movement and breath that they give the mind a needed rest from its day-to-day woes, including the pathological worry caused by an illness.

The Golden Eight Exercises are similar to the Regular Eight Form that has been practiced in China for hundreds of years. I have adapted the regular form exercises to put special emphasis on the heart, the organ of the body that suffers the most in our hectic modern lifestyle. I have also included quotes from *The Yellow Emperor's Classic of Internal Medicine* with each of the eight exercises to help you understand the philosophical underpinnings of Qi Gong.

General Instructions

Do each exercise at least three times, once or twice a day. Stay within your personal comfort level, especially if you are weak or ill. This may mean bending the knees less, not stretching as far, or approximating the movements that are beyond your ability.

Focus on these exercises, keeping your thoughts as tranquil as possible. If your thoughts turn to the stresses in your life, do not dwell on them. Just let the thoughts come and go and focus on form and function.

Proper breathing will help you do this. Keep your breathing smooth, harmonious, and deep while you concentrate on the forms in these exercises. And remember that Qi Gong exercises are done extremely slowly, "as if moving in calm stillness," as an ancient poet described it.

A note of caution: These exercises are usually of great benefit. However, if you develop any problems like extremely sore joints or tendons, then cut back on the amount of exercise you are doing. If the problem persists, consult your doctor.

To Begin: The Natural Standing Form (Figure 8-1)

Each form begins in the Natural Standing Form, which means keeping your feet shoulder-width apart and your back straight and lengthened slightly as if someone were pulling up on a string at the top of your head. Keep your tongue lightly pressed against the roof or your mouth, and your chin slightly tucked in.

Form 1. Reach for Happiness (Figure 8-2)

"After a night of sleep, people should get up early. . . . They should loosen their hair and slow down their movements. By these means they can fulfill their wish to live healthfully."

PURPOSE AND EFFECT: In Chinese medicine, the lungs are the most important organs for creating and sustaining vitality. When we inhale, we take in oxygen and Qi, both of which are vital to our existence. That is why the lung exercises come first in Qi Gong practice.

This exercise has its origin in a famous Buddha statue. He

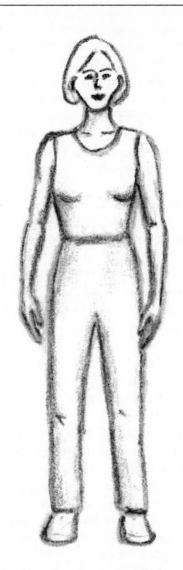

Figure 8-1: The Natural Standing Form

is portrayed with his arms above his head, just as in the exercise. Sometimes he holds a big antique coin, which symbolizes both wealth and the most basic power of life.

The exercise is good for digestive problems; heart, lung, spine, or back problems; and stiff neck and eye problems.

It exercises the entire body through stretching and breathing, also bringing oxygen to the brain for greater alertness. Scientific experiments have shown that inhaling and exhaling with the arms above the head increases lung volume. This exercise decreases the pressure of the internal organs on the heart and increases the venous circulation and blood flow back to the heart. It also massages and tones the internal organs.

When you lock your fingers and push upward, it adjusts and balances your muscles, tendons, skeletal system, nerves, and spine.

When you lower your hands and exhale, you are expelling waste energy and relieving fatigue. At the same time, the abdominal muscles and the diaphragm relax, improving circulation to the abdominal area.

HOW TO BEGIN: From the Natural Standing Form, move your left foot out so your feet are shoulder-width apart. Hands hang relaxed at your sides (a).

As you inhale, gracefully sweep your hands out to your sides, to the front, and then let them settle somewhat in front of the top of your lower *dan tien*, which is located just below your navel. Your palms should be facing up, with the fingers of each hand pointing toward each other (b). As you sweep your hands, imagine that you are gathering up energy and creating a delicate yet powerful ball of energy. Make sure your armpits are open the entire time so the energy flow is not impeded.

Raise your hands, lifting the energy ball very lightly and steadily up to the front of your heart (c). Move slowly, as

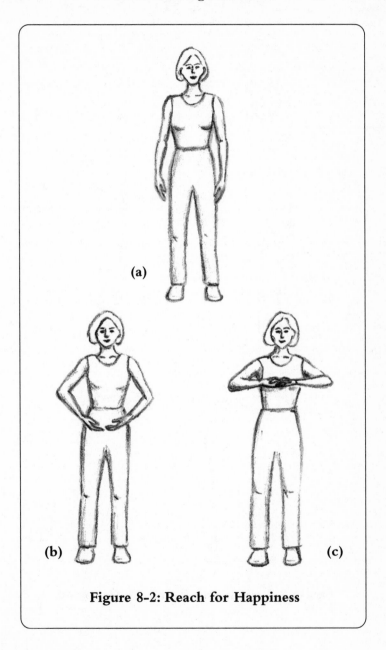

Figure 8-2: Reach for Happiness

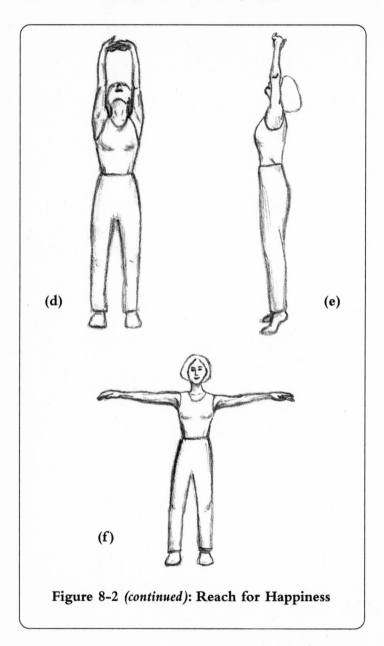

(d)

(e)

(f)

Figure 8-2 *(continued)*: **Reach for Happiness**

though the ball could pop or blow away if you are not gentle and steady in guiding it. Your chest is full and open. (If you have your hands too close to your body, the ball will be squished, and in physical terms, your arms and chest will be constricted.)

Turn your palms down, thumbs rotating inward. Gently interlace the fingers of your opposite hands and lock them together.

As you exhale, with your eyes and head following your hands, raise and rotate your hands (from palms down to palms out front to palms up until they are stretched above your head)(d). Press the ball of energy toward the sky, stretching your arms as far as they can go while keeping your fingers interlocked. Imagine pushing the ball to the far limits of the sky, raising on your toes as far as your balance allows (e). Remain mentally grounded, however, seeing yourself as a rooted tree. Push upward for one second as you fully exhale. Then inhale as deeply as is comfortable.

As you exhale, unlock your fingers and return your head and eyes to a forward position. Let your arms float outward as if gently pushing down two very large balloons (f). Repeat for the desired number of repetitions. When finished, consciously maintain the height and full-chested posture that you have just achieved.

Form 2. The Archer (Figure 8-3)

"The breath of heaven is pure and light."

PURPOSE AND EFFECT: Extending your chest and turning your neck and head improves your circulation, especially in your head and neck area. It also improves heart and lung function. By improving posture and balance, it helps prevent both the structural and functional disorders associated with poor posture.

HOW TO BEGIN: From the Natural Standing Form, move your left foot out so your feet are wider than shoulder-width apart, with your weight evenly distributed. Bend your knees slightly in a horse stance (a). Keep this same foot and knee position throughout the entire exercise.

As you inhale, sweep your arms up into a crossed position about six inches in front of your heart with the right hand inside, palms facing the body.

As you exhale, look at the wrists where they cross. Concentrate on that spot, thinking that you cannot be stopped in your movement. Curl the fingers of your right hand into a loose fist as if to draw the string of a bow. Rotate your left hand so the palm faces away from the left side of the body (b). Imagine that you are holding a bow in your left hand and holding the string with your right hand.

As you inhale, turn your eyes and head to follow the left middle finger while you push the left hand away from the left side of the body until it is fully extended with the hand at a ninety-degree angle from the arm. Visualize this as the left hand pushing a mountain. The right fist "pulls" the string back until the right fist is in front of the right shoulder, with the right, bent arm parallel to the ground (c). The pulling is done with soft, firm strength—not explosiveness.

Allow the hips to rotate partially toward the left hand (thus allowing further lung stretch), and the knees to straighten somewhat. Don't twist your chest. As the arms are at full stretch, concentrate on opening your chest as well as your mind.

As you exhale, return hands to crossed position, continuing to exhale.

Repeat this exercise with the opposite hands.

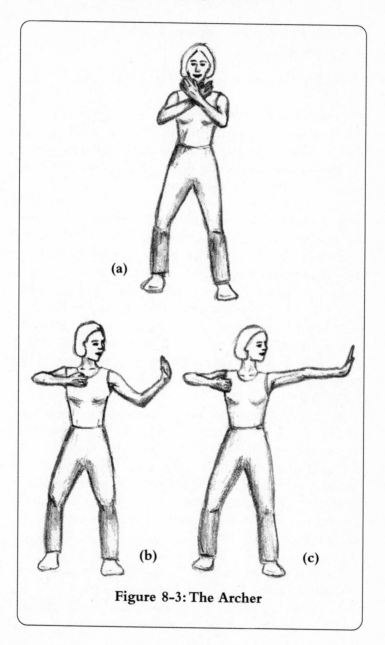

Figure 8-3: The Archer

Form 3. Between Heaven and Earth (Figure 8-4)

"Yin and Yang should be respected to an equal extent."

PURPOSE AND EFFECT: The diametrically opposed movements of the hands pull at and uplift the stomach, spleen, liver, and gallbladder, thus balancing and coordinating them. It also stimulates peristalsis in the digestive system, aiding the stomach and intestines in digestion.

HOW TO BEGIN: Move your left foot to the side so your feet are shoulder-width apart. Sweep your hands out to the sides, to the front, then to an area just below your navel, called the *dan tien*, as though you are gathering energy (a).

As you inhale, bring your hands up in front of your solar plexus (the top part of the stomach, just below the heart).

As you exhale, separate your palms, rotating the right palm upward toward the sky and the left palm downward toward the earth to the side of your body. Go up on your toes if your balance is adequate. Eyes and head follow the movement of the right palm upward.

Move the palms in opposite directions until the right arm is fully extended above the head with the fingers pointing toward the left and the palm facing the sky. The left hand should be fully extended downward with the fingers toward the front and the palm facing the earth (b). Make sure your hands are fully flat and horizontal. If your arms are not flexible enough, you can angle your upper palm somewhat facing forward and your lower palm at less than a full ninety-degree angle from the ground.

Visualize that although the two hands are far apart, they are connected with Qi to both heaven and earth.

As you inhale, return arms to lower rib cage area, placing both palms on the rib cage, fingers facing down (c)

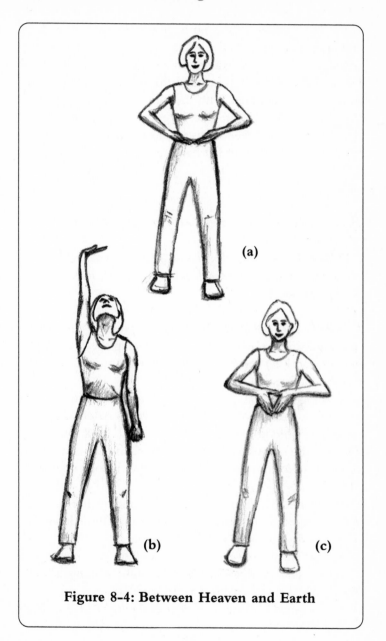

Figure 8-4: Between Heaven and Earth

As you exhale, slide both hands down across your abdomen, ending naturally as far as your hands can go (top of legs), directing bad energy down your torso and out the legs and feet. Return your hands to the starting position in front of your abdomen, with the other palm on top. Repeat the steps for the opposite side. Repeat for desired number of repetitions. (Three repetitions would mean three with right hand up and three with left hand up.)

Form 4. Look Back and Let Go (Figure 8-5)

"They should enable their breath to communicate with the outside world; and they should act as though they loved everything outside."

PURPOSE AND EFFECT: This exercise provides relief from stress and stress-related disorders. Practicing this is especially helpful for long-term stress, emotional turmoil, and the effects of aging.

Turning as far as possible stimulates circulation in the body, neck, eyes, head, and central nervous system, and prevents high blood pressure and eye and neck problems. Twisting the spine stimulates the internal organs and thighs, and is good for the waist. It also improves blood circulation.

HOW TO BEGIN: From the Natural Standing Form, move your left foot out so your feet are wider than shoulder-width apart. Bend your knees in a horse stance.

As you inhale, sweep your hands about five inches out from the side of the waist with thumbs making a well-stretched V and your palms facing down (a).

As you exhale, bend your knees slightly and distribute

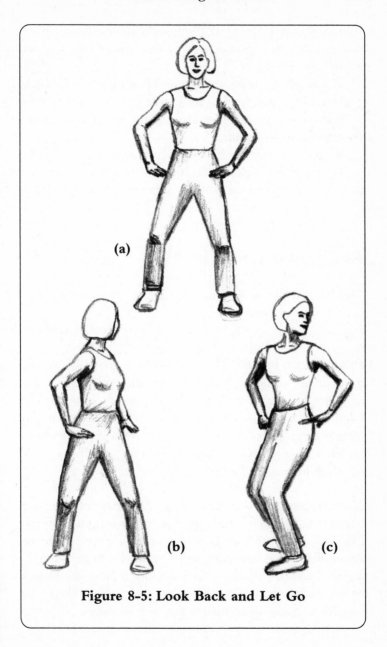

Figure 8-5: Look Back and Let Go

your weight evenly over both feet. As you bend the knees and exhale, guide your energy to your lower *dan tien* (just below your navel).

As you inhale, rotate your upper body to the left as far as possible. Turn your head to look over your left shoulder (b, c). Make sure your shoulders have remained loose. Hold this position for one second.

As you exhale, rotate back to center position.

Repeat in the opposite direction to complete one repetition. Repeat for desired number of repetitions.

Form 5. Twist and Release (Figure 8-6)

"The softness can overcome the stiffness, the calmness can overcome the agitation."

—TAOIST SAYING

PURPOSE AND EFFECT: This exercise has a generally positive effect on the whole body and its circulation of energy. It also relieves tension and can lower blood pressure. In traditional Chinese medicine, twisting the waist helps balance the yin and yang energies of the body, calming the heart and increasing breathing capacity. Many credit this exercise with a tremendous release of anger.

HOW TO BEGIN: Place your left foot so that your feet are wider than shoulder-width apart and your weight is evenly balanced over both feet. Bend the knees slightly in a horse stance. Place your hands on your thighs with thumbs pointing to the rear, with the V between the thumb and fingers widely stretched (a). If you have the strength, bend the knees enough so that your hands can rest near the knees.

Mentally guide your energy down to the soles of your feet and keep it there. In preparation for the next step, make sure your hips and wrists are loose. It is essential to be relaxed in order to obtain benefit from this exercise.

As you inhale, rotate your torso to the left, leading with the left shoulder and looking to the left. Then look to the right and down over your right shoulder, searching to see your right foot (b). (The right shoulder can be lowered slightly, and in all other respects the shoulders have naturally followed the shift of the torso—they do not hunch forward

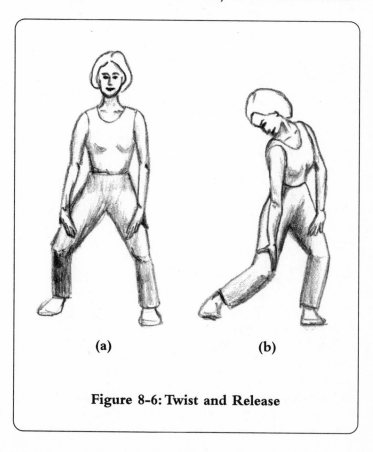

(a)   **(b)**

Figure 8-6: Twist and Release

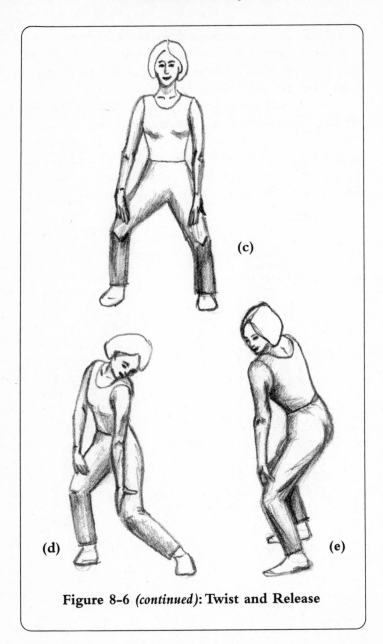

(c)

(d)

(e)

Figure 8-6 *(continued)*: Twist and Release

or pull backward.) As you shift your attention to the right and back, your torso tilts back slightly as if blown by a wind from the front. Imagine a string pulling up on the top of your head at first, and then when you look over your right shoulder, the pull is slightly backward. (This improves your upward energy flow out through your head.) Arch your upper back a little for an extra stretch. It is acceptable to lift the heel of your right foot off the ground. Keep both knees bent. Don't lift any of your fingers off your thighs during the stretch. Hold for one second.

It is very important that the movements be done smoothly, as one long flowing movement. Feel free and flexible throughout, and avoid stiffness in the hips and waist.

As you exhale, bend the right knee and return to the starting position, knees bent (c). Repeat on opposite side to complete one repetition (d, e). Repeat for desired number of repetitions.

Form 6. Bending for Health (Figure 8-7)

"When this force does not support life, its foundation will dissolve."

PURPOSE AND EFFECT: The mind-set during this exercise is that you are gathering the highest-quality energy from heaven and earth as you move. As you gather the best of the best energy, you are nurturing your personal Qi.

The waist and abdominal area are the focus in this exercise. The purpose is to stimulate the kidneys, adrenal glands, and arterial and venous circulation of the lower abdomen. In Chinese medicine, affecting the kidneys can aid the teeth, hearing, and urinary system, including water-retention prob-

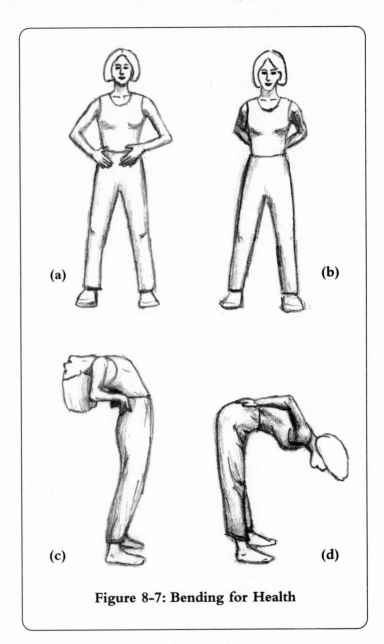

Figure 8-7: Bending for Health

The Golden Eight Exercises

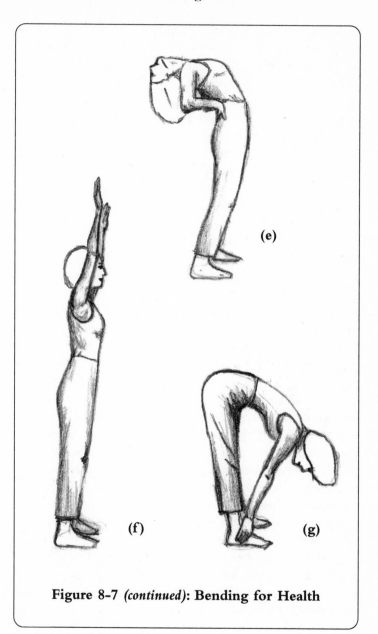

Figure 8-7 *(continued)*: **Bending for Health**

lems. Stimulating the adrenal glands can assist both the urinary and respiratory systems. The solar plexus and lumbar nerve plexus areas are also exercised and stimulated.

When you lean backward, you are guiding energy up from your feet and out of your head. In more physical terms, leaning forward and backward affects blood flow to the brain. It strengthens the nervous system, adjusts overall body metabolism, and improves coordination of the internal organs. This exercise also tones the abdominals, strengthens sexual ability, clears your mind, and brightens your vision. It also helps prostate problems in men and reproductive system problems in women.

CAUTION: People with serious illness, especially heart disease or high blood pressure, should do this exercise lightly and should not bend very far forward or backward.

How to begin: Move your left foot out so feet are a little wider than shoulder-width apart.

As you inhale, sweep your hands to your sides and out front, bringing them close to the abdomen across from where your kidneys are, palms facing abdomen (a).

As you exhale, place your palms on your kidneys (midback), thumbs to the front, fingers pointing to the back (b). Keep your legs fairly straight and your knees loose. (Note: People with hand problems may place the hands lower on the back or buttocks to relieve pressure on the wrist and finger joints.)

As you inhale, lengthen your spine and lean backward as far as is comfortable (c). Try to stretch and bend back all along the spine. Keep in mind that the goal is to straighten and strengthen the spine.

As you exhale, bend forward as far as possible, allowing your head to hang down in front of your body (d). It is important to keep both the waist and the back muscles as soft and relaxed as possible.

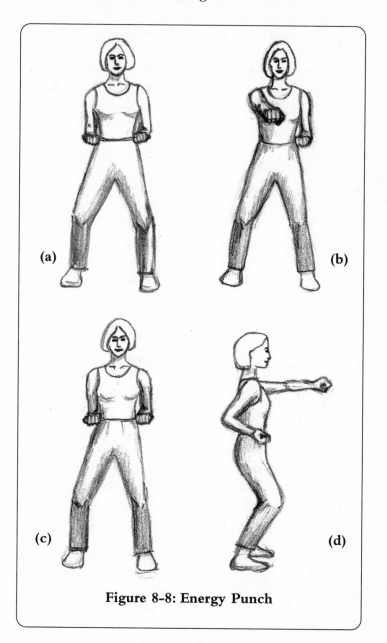

Figure 8-8: Energy Punch

As you inhale, return to a standing position. With your palms on your kidneys again, lengthen your spine and look up and over, leaning backward as far as is comfortable (e).

As you exhale, straighten up, sweeping your arms slightly above and in front of your head (f). Then bend forward as far as is comfortable, making your hands sweep downward without any arm muscle movement. If possible, hold your toes (g). If you can't reach that far, hold your lower legs or knees.

MODIFICATIONS FOR THOSE WITH LOW STAMINA: The breathing can be changed so that every step in this exercise involves both an inhale and an exhale.

Instead of reaching directly for your toes, place your palms (thumbs on inside, fingers on the outside) on your thighs and massage downward to your toes (thus massaging the kidney and liver channels).

Form 7. Energy Punch (Figure 8-8)

"Soul and spirit should be gathered together in order to make the breath of Fall tranquil."

PURPOSE AND EFFECT: This is an emotional exercise that adjusts breathing to increase vitality. It stimulates the central nervous system, lungs, and skeletal and muscular systems, as well as promoting Qi and blood circulation.

HOW TO BEGIN: Move your left foot out so that your feet are a little wider than shoulder-width apart. Do not spread the feet farther apart because you will lose your stable stance. Knees are slightly bent in a horse stance.

As you inhale, sweep your hands, in fists, out to your sides and then out forward, in line with your shoulders.

As you exhale, relax your fists and bring them, palms upward, to the sides of your waist (elbows bent behind)(a). Mentally guide your Qi down into your lower *dan tien*, that area just below the navel. The fists are placed at the sides of the waist so they can carry the Qi from the lower *dan tien*. Imagine an opponent in front of you, and look into his eyes with strong, piercing focus.

As you inhale, punch slowly and forcefully forward, rotating your left fist clockwise so that when the arm is fully extended, the knuckles are on top (palm facing down)(b, d). As you punch, your fist pushes Qi from your body forward. Your mind and the Qi should be one. When you reach full extension, "striking" your imagined opponent with force and confidence, visualize your whole body glowing with Qi in every direction. The fist strikes in the middle of the solar plexus of your opponent. Keep the left shoulder loose and rotate it slightly forward at full extension.

As you exhale, return your fist to the original position (c).

Repeat these steps with the other fist to complete one repetition. Continue for desired number of repetitions.

Form 8. Energy Jump (Figure 8-9)

"Heaven and earth unite to bestow life-giving vigor as well as destiny upon man."

PURPOSE AND EFFECT: The vibrations from landing on your heels go through your spine, helping you open your meridians, stimulating and energizing the nervous system, skeletal system, and blood circulation. This exercise stimulates all the joints of the spine and has a healing effect on spinal problems. It also stimulates the growth of bone marrow and balances the internal organs.

CAUTION: Do not perform this exercise if you have any severe back problems such as a herniated disc.

HOW TO BEGIN: Move your left foot in so your feet are fist-width apart, with your hands at your sides and your back very straight (a). Sweep out your arms to gather energy and then bring your relaxed arms to the sides (b, c).

As you inhale, raise up on your toes, as if pulled by a string, keeping your entire body relaxed like a puppet (d).

As you exhale, imagine that the string is suddenly cut, which makes you drop sharply on your heels (e). Feel the repercussion run up through your back and body. Do your desired number of repetitions.

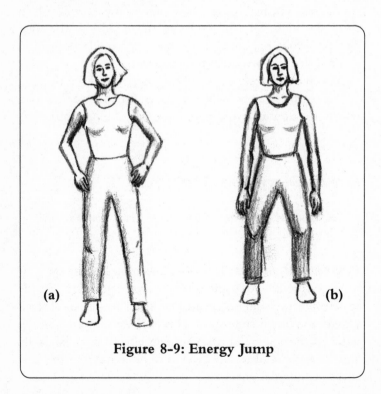

Figure 8-9: Energy Jump

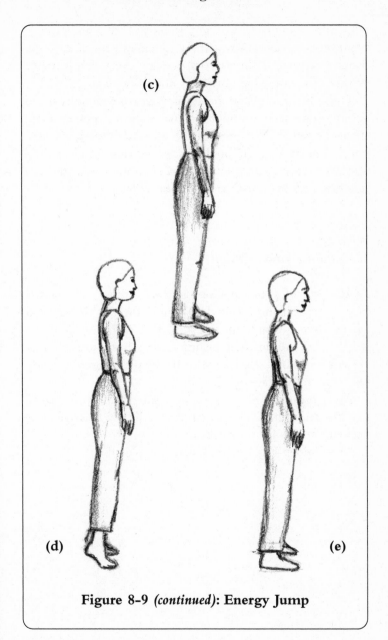

Figure 8-9 *(continued)*: **Energy Jump**

Breathe naturally as you get up on your toes and bounce eight times up and down without touching your heels to the ground. (Unlike the rest of the exercises done in repetitions of three, the bouncing portion is not repeated.)

Finish by placing both hands on your lower abdomen and breathing naturally a minute or two, shutting your eyes and mentally gathering energy in the lower *dan tien* with total concentration. Women should place their right hand on their abdomen covered by their left. Men should place the left hand on abdomen, with right on top of left.

Concluding Your Session

At the end of your Qi Gong session, assume the Natural Standing Form and inhale deeply and slowly, as though you are inhaling a wonderful fragrance that is full of Qi. Then exhale long and slowly, expelling that Qi back into the universe. Focus your mind on your breathing, imagining yourself being fully charged with Qi.

After breathing this way a few times, rub your hands together until they are warm and then lightly massage your face and head with your palms.

The Golden Eight Exercises are completed.

9

AIDS

The first time Samuel realized that his HIV had progressed to AIDS was during a dinner party. As he put food on the plates, he found that he could not hold them straight. Worried that something was happening, he sat down to rest and began slumping uncontrollably to the left. Two days later he was driving to a friend's house when the car began drifting across the center line. He quickly steered it straight, but the car kept "leaning left." Although he blamed the lack of control on the car, he knew that something inside of him was just not right.

A few days later an MRI scan and a brain biopsy revealed the presence of a viral infection on the surface of his brain. Called "PML," this virus sometimes afflicts AIDS patients. When it does, said the neurologist who administered the test, ninety-five percent of the patients die. Of the five percent who live, only five percent regain full use of their bodies.

"I suggest you get your son's affairs in order," the doctor told Samuel's mother. "He has about three months to live."

Samuel deteriorated rapidly after that devastating diagnosis. He lost all use of his left arm and almost all use of his left leg. The left side of his face drooped from lack of control. In essence, the virus had caused a stroke. As Samuel described himself, "I looked like the Elephant Man."

I first saw Samuel at this low point in his life. His mother brought him to my Pasadena clinic, where he sat in silence as I did my diagnosis. By scanning him, I could see other factors besides the brain virus that were contributing to his poor health. His mouth was inflamed with thrush, a fungus common in AIDS patients that starts in the stomach and flourishes in the mouth. I could also see severe blockages in his liver, which would have to be cleared before he could possibly become well.

"Have you taken a lot of drugs?" I asked.

The question surprised Samuel, who did not understand just how I was able to tell that his liver was in such bad condition. "Yes. I snorted cocaine almost daily for fourteen years until I found out that I had this disease," he said. "I did other substances as well. My liver is a mess."

The usual Western treatment for AIDS involves a drug called azidothymidine (AZT), which slows reproduction of the HIV virus and gives the immune system a chance to fight the virus in smaller numbers. This fighting is done by helper T-cells, which engulf the virus and render it helpless.

Eventually, however, the T-cell count drops so low that they cannot adequately fight the AIDS virus. When that happens, the immune system is weakened and opportunistic infections begin to appear, including pneumonia and certain types of cancer. Also common are brain viruses, like the infection that was plaguing Samuel.

My goal was to clear his liver and rid his stomach of the thrush. Both of these problems were toxic to his immune system and were dragging it down, allowing the virus to take over. I told Samuel what I had told others with HIV. "The Chinese believe that when your body gets ill, the sickness creates a bed to lie down on that is inside your body." In Samuel's case, the bed of illness was in large part problems like thrush and the blocked liver.

I explained to him yet another difference between the Western and Eastern approaches to medicine. "When you take the shots and pills of Western doctors, your illness disappears, but the sickness of the Qi surrounding you is still there. When you practice Qi Gong, then the sickness cannot create a bed and grow inside of you. In the case of HIV, Qi Gong makes the immune system function better so disease cannot take hold and further weaken the body."

I performed external Qi treatment on Samuel, with special emphasis on unblocking his liver meridian. I also focused on his spleen, lungs, and kidneys, since Chinese physicians believe that AIDS patients always have blockages in these areas.

I performed external Qi treatments on Samuel every time he came for a patient visit. But I also prescribed herbal medicines and Qi Gong exercises for him to do on his own. I could see the disappointment in his eyes when I began describing the Golden Eight, the exercises I wanted him to do on a daily basis to balance his yin and yang. He was already exhausted from his illness and could not imagine doing any kind of regular exercise.

Still I insisted that he do these exercises. As encouragement, I gave him four reasons why these Qi Gong exercises were important:

- The practice of Qi Gong exercises improves the immune system by increasing lymphocytes and white blood cells in the body as well as the number of antibodies that kill invading germs. This has been shown in research in

China, where a large group of subjects were given blood tests before they began doing regular Qi Gong exercises, and then again after. On the whole, this group showed a greatly enhanced immune system.

- These exercises increase the production of saliva, which contains special antibodies and enzymes that enhance the performance of our immune system.
- The number of T-lymphocyte cells, one of the main measures of immune system health, is increased by Qi Gong exercises. A number of Chinese studies have compared cancer patients who did regular Qi Gong exercises with those who did not. The ones who performed regular exercise had much higher T-cell counts than those who did not. This is of special concern to those afflicted with the HIV virus, since the strength of their immune system is determined by a blood test that counts their T-cells.
- With the practice of Qi Gong—as with all exercise— comes a decrease in the amount of adrenaline in the body, which allows for a slower and healthier metabolism.

"All of these exercises direct your inner energy to kill disease," I said to Samuel. "Even medicine cannot do all of your healing; you have to do some of it for yourself."

I prescribed the Golden Eight exercises to be done approximately thirty minutes per day. He resisted doing such exercises at first, but eventually he managed to do them several times a week.

When that happened, Samuel responded quickly to this traditional Chinese medicine approach. Within three months he was walking without a cane and had regained almost full use of his left hand. His T-cell count, a measure of the strength of the immune system, had risen to 258, from 90 before treatments began (normal is about 1,200). His pain has greatly diminished and his energy has increased.

All of this has pleased Samuel's neurosurgeon, who did not expect to see him alive, let alone walking. "This is amazing," the doctor said to Samuel when he saw him again several months later. "Whatever you are doing, keep doing it."

HERBAL REMEDIES

HIV depletes the immune system, drains the patient of energy, and opens the door to a number of opportunistic infections, most common of which is pneumonia.

There are many Chinese herbal and food remedies that enhance the immune system. Qi Gong treatments focus on the entire body, not just the illness that turns a person into a patient. After all, a weakened immune system can make a person sick, and that illness can in turn make the immune system weaker. That is what I meant when I told Samuel that illness creates a bed inside of the sick person. That bed is largely a weak immune system.

Since AIDS has led to a focus on immune system problems as a contributor to many diseases, I prescribed a number of herbal remedies to increase the strength of the immune system. Although these have special relevance to patients like Samuel who are infected with HIV, these three decoctions for HIV are effective for anyone who needs to boost his or her immunity. I will frequently prescribe one or more of the following decoctions to cancer patients who are taking chemotherapy and are in need of herbal therapy to boost their immune system.

Each of these herbal remedies works on the immune system in different ways. The Bupleurum Decoction is especially effective in raising T-cell counts and is also a good one to use if you are having digestive problems. The Astragalus Root Decoction also elevates T-cell production while it improves liver, spleen, and kidney function. The Dandelion Decoction works well on inflammation and infections in the lungs and the lymph system, which makes it especially effective in fighting flu and nagging colds. Make sure to consider your needs before selecting the one you use.

Bupleurum Decoction

30 grams	Bupleurum (Chai Hu)
24 grams	Scutellaria (Huang Qin)
24 grams	Pinellia (Ban Xia)
12 grams	Fresh Ginger (Sheng Jiang)
18 grams	Ginseng (Ren Shen)
12 grams	Licorice (Gan Cao)
10 grams	Jujube (Da Zao)

Preparation and prescription: Combine all of the herbs together in a pot and cover them with filtered water. Boil this mixture for five minutes and then pour off one cup of liquid for later use. Set this cup aside.

Add another three cups of water to the mixture in the pot and boil until the entire mixture is reduced to about one cup. (Take care not to burn the herbs.) Strain the herbs from the thick tea. Add the cup of tea that was set aside to the thick tea in the pot. This is the herbal remedy.

Drink one of these cups in the morning and the second cup in the afternoon. To prevent stomachache, drink this tea after meals.

How it works: The main purpose of this formula is to increase the immune system, particularly the T-cell count, which is the benchmark of how far the HIV virus has progressed.

One of the best ways to keep immunity high is through the effective digestion of food. To accomplish that goal, I combine bupleurum, scutellaria, pinellia, and ginger. All of these herbs have an effect on the way food is processed by our bodies. Bupleurum, for instance, improves the function of the liver, while ginger settles the acids of the stomach. These herbs also improve the function of the spleen, which is the source of most of our immunity, according to traditional Chinese medicine.

Four of the herbs in this formula—ginger, ginseng, licorice, and jujube—stimulate the functioning of the kidneys, gallbladder, lungs, and liver. These herbs in combination also stimulate the production of T-cells in our bodies. Substantial research conducted on ginseng shows that it alone can improve conditions like anemia, hypertension, ulcers, diabetes, and other conditions, probably due to chemical compounds known as triterpenoid saponins.

In studies in Japan, a formula similar to this one shows great promise as a liver cancer preventative in patients with degenerative liver disease. Used in conjunction with AIDS drugs, it helps improve liver function, largely due to the action of the bupleurum. Another active ingredient in this formula is licorice, which has been shown in research to slow the growth of viruses and bacteria, and help increase the T-cell count.

A Chinese myth about bupleurum, also known as Chai Hu, concerns a worker named Cho Zan, who became so sick with a mysterious fever that the landowner he worked for insisted that he be separated from the other workers. Sick and exhausted, Cho Zan left the farm and collapsed next to a dried-up pond. He made a bed of the reeds surrounding the pond and ate roots that he dug from the damp earth. Gradually, the fever diminished. As he ate more of the roots, he began to regain his strength and energy. Soon he returned to the landowner and asked to have his job back.

"You should be dead," exclaimed the shocked landowner. "What has saved your life?"

Cho Zan thought a moment. "It must have been the roots that I found in the pond's bed," he insisted. "That was the only thing I ate when I was there."

The landowner dispatched workers to collect all of the roots in the pond. Then he began to sell them as a cure for fever and liver ailments. He named this new root after himself (Hu) and the condition it fights in the body, which is heat (Chai).

Astragalus Root Decoction

15 grams	Ginseng
30 grams	Astragalus root (Huang Qi)
15 grams	Pilose Asiabell root (Dang Shen)
9 grams	Atractylodes (Bai Zhu)
6 grams	Licorice root (Gan Cao)
30 grams	Oldenlandia (Bai Hua She She Cao)
30 grams	Rehmannia (Di Huang)
10 grams	Angelica (Dong Quai)
10 grams	Bupleurum (Chai Hu)
10 grams	White peony (Bai Shao Yao)

Preparation and prescription: Combine all of the herbs together in a pot and cover them with filtered water. Boil this mixture for five minutes and then pour off one cup of liquid for later use. Set this cup aside.

Add another three cups of water to the mixture in the pot and boil until the entire mixture is reduced to about one cup. (Take care not to burn the herbs.) Strain the herbs from the thick tea. Add the cup of tea that was set aside to the thick tea in the pot. This is the herbal remedy.

Drink one of these cups in the morning and the second cup in the afternoon. To prevent stomachache, drink this tea after meals.

How it works: This formula elevates the functioning of the immune system by increasing the production of T-cells. It is also extremely effective against common viruses like the flu.

In Chinese medicine, the herbs astragalus, pilose asiabell, and atractylodes are given in combination to increase the activity of the stomach and spleen. This increased activity improves digestion and also acts on the spleen to increase the T-cell count. These herbs are also effective in fighting fungus and bacteria, both of which can gain a dangerous foothold in a person with a weak immune system.

Atractylodes, rehmannia, angelica, bupleurum, and white peony are given in combination to improve the functioning of the liver, lungs, and kidneys. With the improved function of these organs comes a greater ability to clear toxins from the bloodstream, which in turn raises the T-cell count. Part of this effect comes from the improved circulation caused by the Dong Quai, which is known to contain chemicals that cause arteries to dilate, which in turn improves blood circulation.

Licorice and oldenlandia are included in this formula to speed the elimination of toxins from the body.

Medical research confirms the use of astragalus, which is an important ingredient in a number of traditional Chinese remedies. Taken alone as a tonic, it has been found to be an herb that fights cancer and boosts immunity. The effects of this nontoxic herb have been shown in both Eastern and Western studies. A report in *Cancer*, the journal of the American Cancer Society, stated that this herb had strengthened the function of the immune system in a large number of cancer patients who took it.

Its direct effect on cancer has been found in a number of studies.

At Howard University, for instance, researchers combined an extract of astragalus with the drinking water of rats that had lung tumors. Within twenty-four hours, growth in more than eighty percent of the tumor colonies in their lungs had been slowed. The researchers concluded that the herb increased the function of natural killer cells that attack cancer cells. This study has been repeated with the same results at other research facilities.

In studies conducted in China, astragalus has been shown to increase white blood cells in healthy patients as well as in patients with cancer. Another Chinese study showed that it protected against liver damage in patients who were taking chemotherapy. In China, and among certain doctors in the West, it is recommended that astragalus be taken with chemotherapy to reduce the side effects.

Dandelion Decoction

15 grams	Dandelion (Pu Gong Ying)
15 grams	Patriniae Seu Thlaspi (Bai Jiang Cao)
15 grams	Isatis leaf (Da Qing Ye)
15 grams	Isatis Tinctoria (Ban Lan Gen)
15 grams	Indigo (Qing Dai)
10 grams	Dittang (Bai Xian Pi)
6 grams	Rhubarb (Da Huang)
6 grams	Platycodon root (Jie Geng)
15 grams	Honttnynia (Yu Xing Cao)
10 grams	Pomegranate rind (Shi Liu Pi)
10 grams	Phellodendron bark (Huang Bai)
10 grams	Scutellaria root (Huang Qui)

Preparation and prescription: Combine all of the herbs together in a pot and cover them with filtered water. Boil this mixture for five minutes and then pour off one cup of liquid for later use. Set this cup aside.

Add another three cups of water to the mixture in the pot

and boil until the entire mixture is reduced to about one cup. (Take care not to burn the herbs.) Strain the herbs from the thick tea. Add the cup of tea that was set aside to the thick tea in the pot. This is the herbal remedy.

Drink one of these cups in the morning and the second cup in the afternoon. To prevent stomachache, drink this tea after meals.

How it works: This herbal combination reduces inflammation and infection, especially in the lymph nodes and the lungs of AIDS patients. I have also used this to relieve the symptoms of such infectious diseases as mumps and meningitis.

One of the most effective ingredients in this decoction is dandelion. This readily available plant, according to Chinese medicine, eliminates heat and toxins in the blood. Because of that property, it is not uncommon for dandelion to be prescribed for someone with swelling or blood clots. It is also used in the treatment of a number of cancers, especially those of the breast, cervix, and uterus.

Because it has a cleansing effect on the hepatic system, dandelion is effective in relieving jaundice, caused by a liver that is not functioning properly, as is the case with many AIDS patients. It also helps to detoxify a liver that is overloaded with toxins, which makes it an excellent treatment for patients undergoing chemotherapy. Studies in China have compared the blood composition of patients who take dandelion when they are having chemotherapy with those who do not. The results show a higher T-cell count in the dandelion recipients.

Dandelion tonic has many noncancer uses as well. I prescribe it as a means of relieving the pain and symptoms of hepatitis, as well as jaundice and gallstones. It also does wonders for urinary tract infections and pus–producing infections like boils. Because it is high in potassium, heart patients may be prescribed a decoction of this bright flower in China to improve their heart function. It is even recommended in some circles as a remedy for hangover, and I have heard that it is extremely effective in that regard.

Indigo also plays an important role in reducing fever and inflammation. This has long been used by Chinese doctors and American herbalists as a means of reducing swelling in lymph glands, possibly because it stimulates the production and flow of lymph.

FOOD AND DRINK THAT BUILD IMMUNITY

As a means of attacking AIDS through food and drink, I gave Samuel a number of recipes, some of which I have included here.

Licorice Root Tea

A simple but effective method of slowing the growth of HIV is licorice root tea. Japanese researchers have shown that licorice contains substances capable of retarding the growth of the virus.

Licorice also has the ability to reduce fevers and inflammation, most likely because it contains a substance known as glycyrrhizin, which stimulates the adrenal cortex once it is in the body. It also increases the production of bile by the liver and lowers blood cholesterol levels.

Despite the positive effects of licorice, you can get too much of a good thing. When taken in large doses, licorice has been known to cause headaches, raise blood pressure, and cause sodium and water retention.

My advice is to avoid prolonged use of this herb if you

have heart disease, hypertension, or are pregnant. If you feel dizzy or weak, stop drinking this tea immediately.

Preparation and prescription: Add approximately one tablespoon of this sliced herb to a cup of boiling water. Stir and drink.

Main Grain

2 cups	Brown rice
½ cup	Coix (Yi Yi Ren)
½ cup	Soybean (Ta Dou)
½ cup	Chinese green beans
½ cup	Chinese black beans

Preparation and prescription: Combine all five ingredients together in equal portions and soak overnight in filtered water. Add three cups of water and cover the pot. Then bring the mixture to a boil. Reduce heat to a simmer and cook for about forty-five minutes or until it is done. Eat a bowl with every meal.

This was an optional food remedy for Samuel. I do not know if he ate it with every meal, but I do know that it is helpful in whatever quantity it is eaten.

How it works: There has been significant research carried out on the medicinal value of soybeans. In one study published in the *New England Journal of Medicine*, researchers reexamined thirty-eight previous experiments in which soybeans were given to heart disease patients as a means of lowering cholesterol levels. Not only did total cholesterol levels drop an average of nine percent when patients ate soybeans, but the levels of low-density lipoproteins, the particularly bad form of cholesterol, dropped thirteen percent.

Chinese research has shown that soybeans slow the

growth of viruses. This is attributed to a substance called "gray water," which is contained inside of each tiny soybean.

Coix seed is similar to pearl barley, although it's more effective for such medical purposes as regulating water metabolism and eliminating inflammations. It may be obtained at Chinese markets.

Eat this daily for healing purposes.

Creamy Shiitake Mushroom Soup

10 ounces	Fresh Shiitake mushrooms
9 grams	Cordyceps (Dong Chong Xia Cao)
½ cup	Onions, diced
½ cup	Celery, diced
½ cup	Parsley
3 ounces	Potatoes, diced
1 tablespoon	Minced garlic
1½ cups	Chicken broth
⅛ teaspoon	White pepper
¼ teaspoon	Thyme
2 tablespoons	Fresh chopped cilantro

Preparation and prescription: Place all the ingredients in a large saucepan *except* the cilantro. Bring to a boil and then reduce heat. Simmer for fifteen minutes. Place in blender and puree until smooth. Serve immediately, garnished with cilantro.

How it works: The medicinal properties of shiitake mushrooms make them excellent immune system boosters as well as cancer fighters.

Research conducted on shiitake mushrooms in the East and the West have found that it increases the production of T-cells and improves their function, increases the production of interleukin-1, and stimulates macrophages, which protect the body against infection.

Cordyceps, a genus of parasitic fungus found in insect larvae, has been found to suppress coughing and ease asthmatic symptoms.

Samuel's condition improved greatly in a very short period of time. His brain virus almost completely disappeared and he regained his ability to walk. At a time when his doctor said he should be dead, he was beginning to thrive and improve his quality of life.

Curing AIDS is beyond the current scope of medicine, but many of its attendant problems can be addressed best by combining Western and Eastern treatments.

10

Allergies

The Chinese believe that even though the symptoms of allergies manifest themselves in the nose, eyes, and throat, their main cause comes from weakness in the lungs, spleen, and kidneys. When these organs are weak and a change in seasons exposes you to an increase in plant pollens, then the lung energy—or Qi—cannot circulate. When that happens, an allergic reaction takes place.

The view of Western medicine is similar. Western researchers have isolated specific cells in the lungs, intestines, and skin called mast cells. These cells, along with a cell in the blood called a basophil cell, sometimes overreact to foreign bodies like pollen and release too much of the chemical histamine. This causes irritation to different areas of the body. This is why antihistamines are a popular treatment for allergies.

In China, we believe that you are born with allergies to pollen or acquire them later on in life. One of the ways of getting allergies later is through physical or mental stress.

The effects of stress on the human body are extreme.

Medical tests have shown that stress can lower the body's ability to fight a wide variety of diseases, from the common cold to cancer. So it makes sense to me that stress can cause a person to start having allergic reactions. It should come as no surprise to find that the patient in the following case study came down with a severe allergy to a wide variety of pollens. When he told me his story, I told him it was a wonder that his medical problems were so slight.

This patient, whom I will call Wan, went on an expedition into the Devil's Valley. In the Qinren Mountains near the province of Sinkiang, this valley has been known to contain large quantities of gold and draws prospectors from all over the world.

Wan was in one such expedition. He and fourteen fellow prospectors ventured into the valley in search of fortune. As they proceeded into the valley, said Wan, they saw lush meadows with high green grass and bright beautiful flowers that none of them had seen anywhere else. At the entrance to the valley were the remains of ancient stone temples. The valley floor in front of these temples was littered with bones from both animals and humans. The beauty, mystery, and terror of the scene sent a chill through the members of the expedition. For a time they considered stopping right there and returning home. Many people had disappeared while searching for gold in that valley. Rumors abounded as to why. Some blamed wild animals. Others blamed these disappearances on poisonous plants.

But after a brief conference, they decided to press on in search of gold. The first day of the hike went well. Wan and the rest of the group were awestruck by the beauty that surrounded them. The high mountains and the roaring river piqued their senses; the cool air and flatness of the valley made hiking easy.

On the second day, Wan was at the rear of the group as

they walked through a field of chest-high grass. Suddenly the fourteen people ahead of him dropped into the ground. Slowly and carefully he approached the spot where they had disappeared. To his horror he realized that they had been hiking on an underground river. The fourteen explorers ahead of him had fallen through a thin layer of earth and were swept away by the water below.

Wan began to shake with fear. Suddenly he was alone in a valley that could suck him underground and drown him as it had his friends. For the rest of the day and night he did not move. It was not until the afternoon of the next day that he began to crawl back through the valley, testing the ground as he went to see if it would hold him or collapse into the river below.

His return trip took several days. Savage lightning storms swept the valley almost daily. Nearby trees were split by lightning bolts. When he finally reached the stone temples at the entrance to the Devil's Valley, he was wet, frightened, and deeply exhausted.

After that he was afflicted by a severe case of allergies, which manifested themselves with the classic symptoms of sneezing, itchy eyes, and respiratory problems. That was when he came to see me at my office in Shanghai.

I was fascinated by Wan's story and somewhat surprised that he did not come down with something far more serious than allergies. Stress like that could have made him sick in any number of ways, I told him. Developing allergies was a small price to pay compared to what might have happened.

I gave him several external Qi treatments to clear the blockages in his spleen and kidneys, which in turn helped clear the fluid that had accumulated in his lungs. Then I gave him the following exercises and herbal formula to relieve the symptoms of his allergies.

Playful Exercises to Open the Lungs
(Figures 10-1, 10-2, 10-3)

Lean against a wall with your hands shoulder-width apart and your feet about three feet from the wall (Figure 10-1). Push against the wall as hard as possible, so that you can feel the pressure building in your shoulders. Hold this position for a few seconds.

With your hands held much wider than your shoulders, lean against the wall and push as hard as possible until you feel the pressure in the middle of your chest (Figure 10-2). Hold for a few seconds.

With your hands held over your head, lean against the wall and push as hard as possible so you feel the pressure on your back, behind your shoulders (Figure 10-3a, b). Hold this position for a few seconds.

PURPOSE AND EFFECT: Repeat these movements six times. Effects should be felt almost immediately. In addition to opening the lung meridians, this exercise brings blood to the chest and lungs and opens the air sacs in the lungs that have likely clamped down due to the allergic reaction.

These exercises are also good for children who are afflicted with allergies because they have the element of play in them.

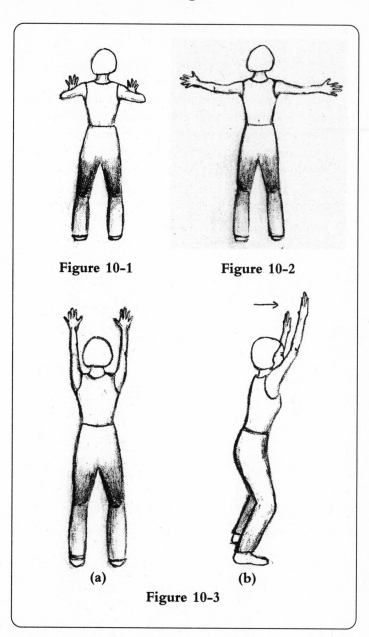

Figure 10-1   Figure 10-2

(a)   (b)

Figure 10-3

Sinus Massage (Figures 10-4, 10-5)

Massage the sides of your nose with your index fingers, up and down, thirty-six times (Figure 10-4).

With your index fingers, find the meridian points located between the corner of your eyes and your nose (Figure 10-5a). Run your fingers across the top of each eye and back again (b), thirty-six times. Then repeat these motions across the bottom of your eyes, thirty-six times.

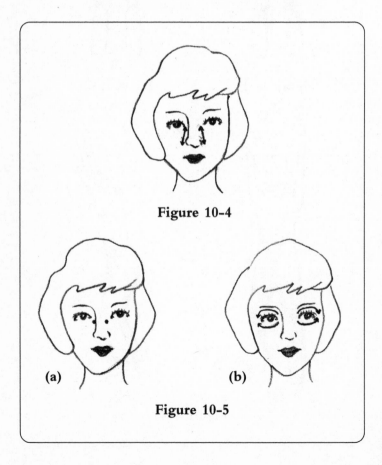

Figure 10-4

(a)   (b)

Figure 10-5

PURPOSE AND EFFECT: The sinus cavities become so swollen by allergies that they lose their ability to eliminate mucus. These massages not only reduce swelling of the sinus tissue, they also help clear mucus from the airways.

HERBAL REMEDIES

In Shanghai, where air pollution is bad and the number of allergy cases is high, I was summoned to the home of a high government official to treat her child's allergy to the bad air.

I prescribed an herbal remedy and recommended a dietary plan for the boy to follow. But he needed Qi Gong exercises as well, so I prescribed the exercises just given. I devised a method of play that would be fun for the child and effective as an exercise treatment for his asthma.

I had the mother face the child and hold his hands. Then I told her to "wrestle" with the boy, having him push against her hands, first at shoulder-width, then much wider than the shoulders, and finally with his hands fully extended over his head. These playful push-aways opened lung meridians that made it easier for him to breathe.

Adults can also use a partner if they wish. However, it is usually easier to perform these exercises against a wall. Whichever method you choose, however, the results of these exercises are excellent.

Using these exercises and the following herbal remedies, it took the little boy in Shanghai about a week to start sleeping throughout the night without wheezing. Most of my patients in the United States experience fast relief as well.

Allergy Antidote

15 grams	Honeysuckle (Jian Yin Hua)
15 grams	Acorus Rhizome (Shi Chang Pu)
15 grams	Xanthium fruit (Kang er Zi)
12 grams	Scutellaria root (Huang Qin)
12 grams	Eucommia bark (Du Zhong)
9 grams	Ephedra (Ma Huang)
9 grams	Asarum (Xi Xin)
9 grams	Astragalus root (Huang Qi)
9 grams	Siler (Fang Feng)
9 grams	White Atractylodes (Bai Zhu)

Preparation and prescription: Combine all of the herbs in a large pot and cover with filtered water. Boil for three minutes until it has the color of dark tea. Pour the tea through a strainer and into a container and keep it in the refrigerator.

Drink a glass of the tea each day for five days and then skip two. Follow this routine for one month.

How it works: In traditional Chinese medicine, honeysuckle, acorus rhizome, and xanthium fruit are combined to open the nasal passages. It does this through an antihistamine effect that slows the production of mucus in the sinuses. These herbs also relive the itching eyes that are associated with allergic reactions.

In treating allergies, the air passageways of the lungs must also be opened. To do that, I combine scutellaria root, eucommia bark, and ephedra. These herbs open the air sacs of the lungs that clamp down in the course of allergy problems. By opening these air sacs, the patient can breathe much more freely.

The most active of these ingredients is the ephedra, which has been used for thousands of years in China as a means of opening the airways of the lungs. This makes it an effective herbal for asthma and hay fever as well as allergies. The effective portion of this herb is thought to be the alkaloids present in its leaves and stems.

Opening the air passages is only dealing with the surface effects of allergies. The Chinese believe that to treat allergies completely, you must also treat the kidneys and liver. To treat these organs, I combine astragalus root, siler, and white atractylodes. These herbs improve the immune system to help fight off allergies, and they also open the pores of the skin to release the bad energy caused by the allergies.

Astragalus is one of the oldest and most famous of all Chinese herbs. Western research has shown that it does indeed improve the immunity of those who take it, which supports the Chinese view of this herb. In China it is frequently taken as a way of fighting off persistent colds.

There is a beautiful myth about honeysuckle that provides poetry to the workings of this formula's main ingredient.

In ancient China, a couple had twins that were loved by everybody. The parents named them Silver Blossom and Golden Blossom. Growing up they were very close, so close that they did not want to marry because they would have to live in separate households.

"We want to live together and be buried together," the two girls told their parents. "We never want to be apart."

In the winter of her twentieth year, Golden Blossom became extremely sick. A doctor came and told her parents that death was imminent.

"She has heat poison fever," said the doctor. "There is nothing I can do for her."

Silver Blossom stayed by Golden Blossom until she died. Then Silver Blossom, too, became very ill with the fever. In a short period of time she died.

The parents buried their beloved twins together on the banks of a beautiful lake.

By the end of spring, a flower blossomed on the grave site that turned from white to gold. The town doctor used this flower on a patient with a fever and found that it cured the affliction. He tried it on a person with allergies and found that it cured his affliction as well.

The doctor picked many of the plants and gave them to other physicians. When they asked him what it was called, he said "Jian Yin Hua," which means golden and silver flowers, which is the way the Chinese say honeysuckle.

FOODS THAT FIGHT ALLERGIES

As an added boost to healing, I recommend the following recipes to my patients with allergies. As I told Wan, my frightened patient, "Foods can alleviate as well as cause allergies. If you choose the right ones, you can help reverse your reactions." He and other allergy patients have received considerable relief from the food remedies that follow.

Cordyceps Allergy Relief

½ ounce	Cordyceps (Dong Chong Xia Cao)
½ ounce	Glehnia (Sha Shen)
¼ ounce	Ginger
3 ounces	Salted pork or ham (sliced)
8 ounces	Fresh white fish or chicken
4 cups	Water

Preparation and prescription: Combine the ingredients in a steamer and cook for one hour. Add salt and pepper and cooking wine, if you wish, for additional flavor.

How it works: In addition to removing tightness from the lungs, which is a function of cordyceps and ginger, the glehnia makes this dish a good purifier for the kidneys and blood.

Lotus Seed Cough Remedy

2 ounces	Lotus seeds
2 ounces	Chinese lily bulb (Bulbus Lilii) (Bai He)
¼ ounce	Ginger (thin-sliced)
½ pound	Lean pork (sliced)
3 cups	Water
3 pieces	Scallion

Preparation and prescription: Combine the ingredients in a large pot and simmer together for ninety minutes until the lotus seeds are soft enough to eat. Add salt and pepper and cooking wine to taste.

How it works: Besides contributing its wonderful taste, ginger contains chemicals known as cardiotonics, which are known to have anti-coughing properties and also function as painkillers. Lotus seeds add an exotic sweetness to this dish while acting as a stimulant to the kidneys, which have blocked energy when a person is experiencing allergies.

Sweet Cough Remedy

1 teaspoon	Fritillary powder (Bei Mu)
1 teaspoon	Caterpillar fungus (Dong Chong Xia Cao)
1 cup	Ginkgo seed (Bai Guo)
¼ cup	Red dates
1 teaspoon	Lycium fruit (Gou Qi Zi)
1 teaspoon	White peony (Bai Shao Yao)
2 halves	Pears
⅛ cup	Rock sugar or honey
2½ cups	Water

Preparation and prescription: Soak the ginkgo in warm water for two hours, then peel off the shells. Boil two cups of water in a pot and add fritillary powder, caterpillar fungus, ginkgo seeds, and lycium fruit. Cook for ten minutes over medium heat and add pears (cut into pieces) and the sugar or honey. Cook for five minutes and serve.

How it works: This recipe equals a single dose, which can be taken as often as three times per day after every meal. It is especially effective in relieving severe coughs as well as bronchitis and asthma.

These treatments were very effective for Wan and the little boy, as they are for so many allergy sufferers. The herbal remedies are very good at lessening the severity of the allergies, but I think the Qi Gong exercises produce some natural antihistamine chemicals internally that bring the body back into balance.

For Wan, as for many people, allergies are a long-term—if not lifetime—problem, no matter what course of medical treatment is chosen. This Qi Gong method of treatment allow for a natural approach to relief, which should be pursued especially during allergy season or whenever you have an allergy attack.

11

Arthritis

Where Qi Gong masters gather, patients are sure to follow. That was the case in 1988, at the annual meeting of the Qi Gong Science Research Association, held near Canton. Wealthy businessmen and famous people came from all around the Pacific Rim to seek healing for their illnesses.

At one point in the conference I was approached by the head of the Xinhua News Agency, the governmental organization in charge of the reclamation of Hong Kong. His problem was a minor one that I was able to treat quite easily. Nonetheless, his wife was present for the healing and was quite impressed. She pulled me aside and asked if I could perhaps provide healing for the famous Ms. Ku.

Without hesitation I said yes.

Ms. Ku was the Queen of Chinese Folk Dancers. Her beauty and grace was renowned throughout China. Treating her would be similar to working with a star like Madonna in this country.

"What is her problem?" I asked the woman.

"Arthritis," came the reply.

In Western medicine, arthritis is treated with a variety of drugs, exercises, and therapies. Common recommendations involve treatment with heat lamps and hot water. Some Western physicians recommend exercises to keep the joints nimble, and some even suggest that people with bad arthritis move to a warm, dry climate.

Medications are used as well. Many arthritis patients take daily doses of aspirin or other anti-inflammatory drugs. If that does not work to reduce pain, they may be given injections of cortisone directly into the joint. Although drugs like cortisone will almost certainly provide temporary relief, they often lead to joint destruction in the long term.

In China, arthritis is believed to be the result of the body being invaded by cold and damp. This can happen in a number of different ways. For example, working too long and hard in bad weather can lead to exhaustion and make the joints susceptible to the effects of the cold and damp.

Because of this concern about cold and damp, there is a folk tale that warns against making love outside, particularly at the beach, high in the mountains, during a thunderstorm, or in a temple. It is in these places that cold and damp energy can invade the body through the pores that have become open due to the excitement and ecstasy. Although I had heard this warning about sex on many occasions, I had never encountered it as a cause of this common illness.

That changed when I met Ms. Ku.

That evening I was introduced to the beautiful Ms. Ku. She was dressed like a Hong Kong fashion model, her slim figure sheathed in a white silk dress. She was wearing flat shoes, which was the first hint that she was having trouble with her feet. (Most fashionable Hong Kong women wear high heels in public.) Another clue was the long black gloves she wore. It was warm this time of year, and I felt that she wore these gloves to conceal something from the adoring fans who gathered around her.

We were taken to a private room at a nearby hotel by the government official's wife, who then left us alone. I asked Ms. Ku to sit down and I immediately began to scan her, using the powers of external Qi to diagnose the extent of her problems. What I saw hurt me. Bad energy pervaded every joint in her hands and feet. Even though she smiled warmly, I could tell that she was experiencing incredible pain that made it difficult even to move her fingers and toes.

I asked her to remove her shoes and gloves, which reaffirmed my diagnosis. They were becoming disfigured, beginning to curl up like claws. Her calf muscles were shrinking and her knees had begun to swell. As I examined her, she began to weep. Chinese dance is a language of beauty that is conveyed through intricate movements of the hands and feet. Now that beauty was being taken away from her. Could I help her? she asked anxiously.

I had her lie down on the bed and close her eyes. "Please relax your entire body and think about the bottom of your feet," I said. Then I began to administer external Qi Gong therapy. I started by putting my left hand about five inches above her head. I then passed my right hand from her forehead down toward her feet, giving her the Qi energy necessary to open her meridians and allow the dampness and coldness to leave her body. Her face began to twitch as I did this and then she began to cry as her pent-up emotions came out.

"I want to tell you why I think this has happened to me," she said.

As a dancer, said Ms. Ku, she was constantly rehearsing. It was not uncommon for her to rise early in the morning and practice a variety of dances and moves until late at night. These practice sessions weakened her both physically and emotionally. Despite the fact that she was a famous dancer, she had almost no social life because of these practice sessions. She was a married woman, but still she had no private life. It seemed as though her entire life consisted of either performing onstage or preparing to perform. Practicing left her with little energy.

It was during these practice sessions that a wealthy man from Hong Kong began showing up. He was a great fan of hers and wanted to watch her as much as possible, even during practice. She enjoyed the attention. The man was handsome and rich and easy to talk to. Soon he began to ask if she would accompany him to dinner. At first she said no, feeling that anything that distracted from her dancing was not good. Eventually, however, her need for companionship took over and she agreed to go to a late-night dinner with him.

As they drove across the city, their passions began to swell and they decided to stop in a park and make love. Even though it was a cold night, they lay on the ground and made passionate love. They lay together until the chill in their bones forced them to return to the car. After that night, said Ms. Ku, she began to ache in all of her joints. From then on, the pain had increased until she could barely dance at all. Now her greatest fear was not that she would never dance again, but that she would become physically incapacitated for life.

I listened to the rest of her intriguing story as I pulled all of the damp and cold energy from her body that I could. Had a single tryst in the park really done such damage to this great dancer? Did this act of infidelity lead to such deep psychological guilt that it began to affect her physically? Had the mind led the body, or had the body led the mind into this dilemma? I asked myself these questions as I forced the bad energy from several meridian points.

After about fifteen minutes of treatment, I asked her to stand up. "Move your fingers, legs, and feet," I said to her.

As she followed my instructions, she began to smile. "My pain is gone!" she exclaimed with delight.

I knew I had provided only temporary relief. Arthritis pain is devious, I told her. Sometimes treatment makes it go away but it comes back. "This type of sickness takes a long time to heal," I told Ms. Ku. "You must commit yourself to recovery."

I prescribed specific exercises to help remove the cold and damp energy from the body as well as improve the strength and flexibility of her joints and muscles. I also prescribed herbal remedies formulated to rid the body of excess "cold" and "damp," and to encourage the healing process.

SPECIAL EXERCISES FOR ARTHRITIS

In addition to the Golden Eight Exercises, I prescribed two special exercises for Ms. Ku. I learned these exercises myself from a Taoist master who was introduced to me by Master Kwan. He was a remarkable man, who looked to be in his sixties.

When I discovered his true age (one hundred and eight), I was both shocked and excited. "How do you stay so young?" I asked.

"Flexibility," he responded. "I have made sure to lose none of my flexibility over the years."

Every day, he did an exercise routine that resembled the Golden Eight Exercises. This kept him young until he was well into his eightieth year. After that, however, he began to feel twinges of arthritis. It was then that he developed the following exercises, their goal being to combat arthritis.

"Fight illness from the first day it arrives," said the Taoist master. "That way it is less likely to grow."

I couldn't disagree with someone one hundred and eight!

Massage of the Fingers (Figure 11-1)

Place your right hand in your left. Using the thumb and forefinger of your left hand, squeeze the joints of your pinky finger one at a time, applying pressure and bending them back as far as comfortable (Figure 11-1a, b, c). As you move higher up the finger, slowly raise your right elbow until it is above your shoulder. Lower it when you have reached the end of your finger.

Repeat this three times with each finger and thumb of the right hand. Then follow the same procedure with the left hand.

PURPOSE AND EFFECT: Squeezing and bending the finger joints improves their flexibility and strength, which are two factors that diminish with arthritis. Raising the elbow is very important in this exercise as well, since there are three major Qi channels above and below the arm that are connected to all of the organs. By raising your elbow as you massage the joints of your fingers, you are stimulating your internal organs as well.

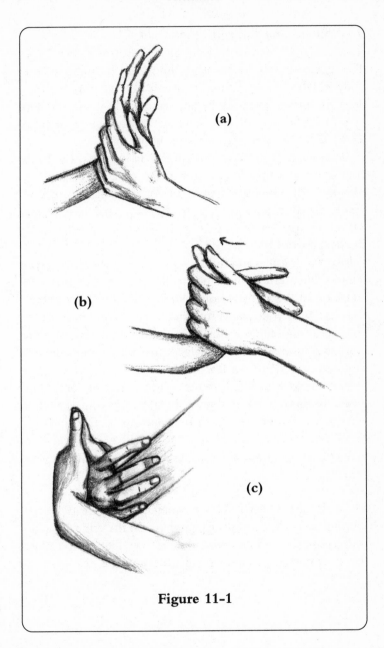

(a)

(b)

(c)

Figure 11-1

The Swimming Dragon (Figure 11-2)

This gyrating exercise involves almost all the joints of the body, much as a swim through a cold lake would involve a dragon's entire body. To begin, stand with your feet and knees together and your palms together in a prayer fashion (a). Hold your tongue against your upper palate.

With your palms together prayer fashion, slowly bend your knees and thrust your hips to the right as you look to the right (b). Hold for a short period of time and reverse directions, thrusting your hips to the left as you look to the left (c). Thrust four times with each hip before moving on to the next part of the exercise.

Bend your knees and hold your palms together in a prayer fashion. Then raise your hands to the left side of your head and look to the right as you thrust your hips in that direction (d). With your palms together, draw a half circle under your head and across your chest to the right side of your body and hold your hands parallel to your shoulders (e, f). Hold that position for a few seconds.

Next, hold your hands straight out in front of you, palms down. With your knees slightly bent, sweep your arms left and right five times as you thrust your hips in the direction opposite to your arms (g, h, i).

Repeat the entire Swimming Dragon movement four times.

PURPOSE AND EFFECT: This movement works nearly every joint in the body, with special emphasis on the spine. In addition to improving joint strength and flexibility, these movements stimulate the kidneys and adrenal glands.

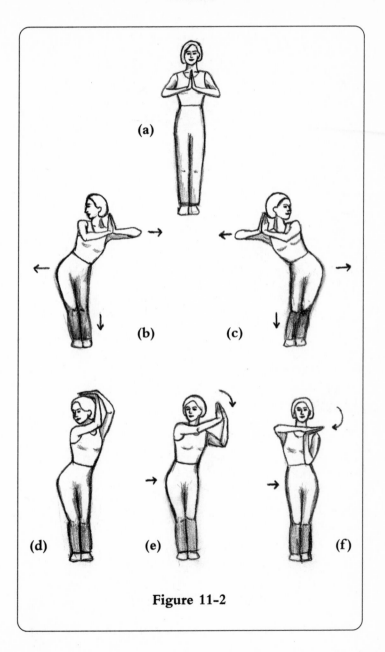

Figure 11-2

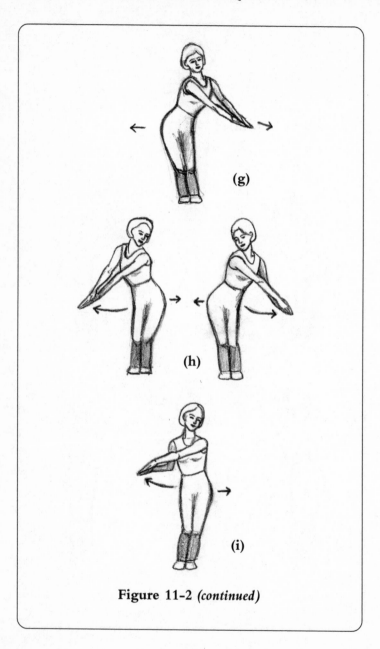

Figure 11-2 *(continued)*

HERBAL REMEDIES

Traditional Chinese medicine has a number of effective remedies for arthritis. Those following are among the best, since they attack the pain and swelling that are the cause of discomfort in this disease.

First Herbal Formula

15 grams	Stephania root (Fang Ji)
15 grams	Rehmannia (prepared) (Shen Di)
9 grams	Cinnamon twig (Gui Zhi)
9 grams	Siler (Fang Feng)
9 grams	Licorice root (Gan Cao)
30 grams	Notopterygium root (Qiang Huo)
30 grams	Dandelion (Pu Gong Ying)

Preparation and prescription: Combine all the herbs together in a pot and cover with five cups of water. Boil until they become a thick tea and then pour through a strainer. Drink one glass three times a day for five days and then stop for two days. Repeat this cycle for one month.

How it works: In traditional Chinese medicine, arthritis is thought to be caused by a body that has become somehow weakened and has let the cold and damp in. In my experience, I have found that women are more likely to get arthritis, probably because they have menstrual periods that lower their immunity on a monthly basis, while a man has a fairly constant level of immunity. Combine this factor with the stresses of modern living, and you have an increased susceptibility to diseases like arthritis that are strongly linked to the immune system.

This herbal formula rids the joints of excessive heat or dampness and cold and is recommended for painful arthritis.

The main ingredients in this formula are the stephania root and the rehmannia. In Chinese medicine these herbs are prescribed to get rid of damp and cold. Rehmannia especially is a favorite in some tonic formulas because of its ability to take the pain out of joints by getting rid of excess fluid in the body.

Cinnamon adds warmth to the body by improving circulation. I think that effect is caused by an oil called cinnamic aldehyde that is contained in the bark of this tree. To experience this effect, you might try chewing on a cinnamon stick, which can be purchased in most any supermarket. Not only will you experience the circulation–enhancing properties of this herb, you will also feel its heat on your tongue and the pleasure of its pungent taste and smell. In addition to providing arthritis relief, the oil from cinnamon contains antibacterial properties and is used in the Orient as a means of controlling such bacteria as *E. coli,* staph, and thrush.

Licorice root is also a potent portion of this formula, and in many other traditional Chinese formulas. Not only does it improve the taste of many herbal remedies, licorice works as a laxative and sedative and is even used at times to ease stomach ulcers. Many cultures have used licorice in medicines, and the herb has even been found in the excavated tombs of Egyptian pharaohs. It may be effective against arthritis because of the recent revelation by Chinese and Japanese chemists that licorice stimulates the production of interferon, an antiviral substance produced by the body's cells.

Because it contains glycyrrhetinic acid, which acts like aspirin, licorice also takes some of the pain caused by arthritis out of the joints.

Last but not least I mention dandelion, another of the all-purpose remedies of Chinese medicine. Because it contains a number of chemicals, vitamins, and minerals, dandelion is used for a wide variety of ailments. It has anti–inflammatory properties that make it especially useful in fighting arthritis.

It can also be used as a cure for constipation. And it stimulates the liver to produce more bile and can even be applied topically to remove some types of warts. It also has diuretic effects, which makes it good as a blood cleanser as well as a tonic for arthritis. It is these blood-cleansing effects that make dandelion the stuff of Chinese legend.

As myth has it, dandelion (Pu Gong Ying) first came to public attention in ancient China when the daughter of a high official developed a painful lump on her left breast. The pain was so tremendous that the young girl began to cry in her bedroom. This brought her mother, who misunderstood the nature of the swelling and accused her daughter of being pregnant. Distraught and in pain, the daughter decided to commit suicide. She walked down to the river at night and jumped into the water in hopes of drowning.

At that moment, a fisherman named Pu, who was night fishing with his daughter, rowed to her rescue. When they pulled the girl into the boat, she told them why she wanted to die.

"I can heal your problem," said Pu.

They rowed to the fisherman's home, where he boiled some flowers that he had picked from the mountainside. Then he poured the water into a cup and had the young girl drink it.

After she had drunk this tea for a few days, the girl's pain and swelling was gone. The fisherman took her home to her grateful parents, who realized that they had misjudged their daughter.

"How did you heal her?" they asked the fisherman.

When he showed them the flower, they decided to give it a name that would honor both the fisherman (Pu Gong) and their daughter (Gong Ying).

The name has stayed the same ever since.

Second Herbal Formula

| 4 ounces | *Aristolochia Millissima* Hance (Xuan Gu Feng) |
| 16 ounces | Rice wine |

Preparation and prescription: Combine the herb and the liquor in a bottle or decanter and let the concoction sit for one month. When it is ready, drink half a shot glass of the liquor twice a day, for one month.

How it works: Herbs and alcohol that gain medicinal properties when they are combined are called tinctures. In this particular tincture, the aristolochia warms the joints and reduces the pain. It also acts as a diuretic to help get rid of excess fluid that sometimes accumulates around the joints and reduces their range of motion.

CAUTION: Because this formula contains alcohol, do not drive or operate machinery after it has been consumed. Also, so not exceed the recommended dosage. This formula is not recommended for anyone with a history of substance abuse.

HEALING MEALS FOR ARTHRITIS

In addition to the exercises and herbs, I would like to have given Ms. Ku some dietary advice as well. At the time that I treated her, she was so busy that she seldom had time to devote to "eating from the medicine cabinet," as I put it. Had she been willing, I would have prescribed her a number of foods and dishes, including the recipe that follows.

Sautéed Beef with Herbs

¼ ounce	Acanthopanax root bark (Wu Jia Pi)
¼ ounce	Eucommia bark (Du Zhong)
1 pound	Flank steak, sliced thin
1	Carrot, sliced and steamed
1 bunch	Spinach
1 clove	Garlic, minced
2 ounces	Ginger
2 tablespoons	Cooking wine
½ teaspoon	Honey
2 tablespoons	Cornstarch
2 tablespoons	Soy sauce
5 tablespoons	Sesame oil

Instructions: Combine the herbs in a pot with two cups of water and boil down to one-quarter cup of juice. Remove the herbs.

Marinate the beef in the wine, soy sauce, honey, cornstarch, and herb juice.

Heat the sesame oil to a high temperature in a skillet and brown the garlic and ginger. Then add the beef and the cooked carrot and stir-fry until the beef is cooked to your liking.

Heat sesame oil to a high temperature in another skillet and add the spinach. Cook for thirty seconds.

Combine the spinach and the beef in a bowl and serve.

How it works: Since arthritis is considered an invasion of cold and damp in Chinese medicine, we recommend foods that dispel wind and dampness while strengthening the bones and sinews at the same time. In this recipe, acanthopanax root acts as a diuretic to dispel fluid in the body that has built up in the joints. Eucommia bark is included to improve the function of the kidneys and liver. It also works as a painkiller, and is especially effective in relieving pain in the lower back and the knees.

I think prevention is one of the most important strategies for arthritis. It is important to act as soon as signs of arthritis manifest themselves. A person who has sore joints or chronic stiffness should begin exercises and herbal treatments immediately. Had Ms. Ku done that, she would not have missed a day of dancing.

Several years later, by the way, I saw Ms. Ku in Los Angeles. My wife and I were dining at a restaurant in Chinatown when I saw her at a nearby table. Her beauty and fame made her the center of attraction. Everyone was looking at her, as was I. She had no gloves on this time and her hands looked elegant and supple. She was wearing high heels and walked with no pain, only the grace of a dancer.

At one point I caught her eye, but she turned away quickly. At first I felt hurt. Then I realized why she did not want to see me. The man she was with was not her husband! His presence with her in Los Angeles would have been difficult to explain.

We toasted across the room and let it go at that.

12

Prostate Cancer

There are more than one hundred types of cancer, caused by factors ranging from genetic defects and low immunity to air pollution, poor diet, radiation, tobacco, and industrial chemicals. Because there are so many different types of cancer, it is impossible for me to offer treatments in this book for each and every one. Instead I will present the prostate case study that I discussed in chapter seven to give you an idea how Chinese doctors treat cancer.

Like Westerners, the Chinese have many different approaches to cancer. As a cancer specialist at the Red Cross Hospital in Shanghai, I had a great deal of experience in combining the allopathic medicine of the West with Qi Gong and other forms of traditional Chinese medicine. When cancer patients come to me for help, they are sometimes surprised that I recommend combining Chinese medicine with such approaches as chemotherapy and radiation. I find that Chinese and Western medicines combine nicely to attack cancer, like they do other diseases.

There are many studies that confirm the effectiveness of herbal remedies against cancer. Recent studies in the United States concern the bark of the yew tree, which yields a substance known to fight forms of breast cancer. In research conducted worldwide, various herbs have been shown to:

- Kill tumor and other types of cancer cells
- Protect against cancer-causing agents
- Increase the level of anticancer enzymes in the blood
- Protect against damage to healthy tissue caused by radiation treatments and chemotherapy
- Improve liver function in cancer patients
- Boost the function of the immune system

Much research also supports the effectiveness of Qi against cancer. Clinical trials conducted by myself and other researchers have found that external and internal Qi Gong techniques alone can kill cancer cells, increase immunity, improve vitality, and prolong the length and quality of life of a cancer patient. For example:

- External or emitted Qi has inhibited or killed leukemia cancer cells in animals. It has also slowed the growth of melanoma metastasis in animals that were injected with melanoma cancer cells.
- Qi Gong has been shown to speed recovery from surgery as well as chemo and radiation therapies.
- Qi Gong can shrink cancerous tumors, as proven by X rays taken before and after Qi Gong therapy. It also increases survival rates of cancer patients.
- The health of the immune system improves with Qi Gong. Studies have shown that Qi can help increase white blood cell counts. It can also stabilize them, keeping the

important cells from dropping dangerously low during chemotherapy and other forms of treatment.

Cancer must be fought intelligently and on every front. As I tell my cancer patients: "Make your fight against this disease a full-time job. Use the arsenals of both Western and Eastern medicine. Include everything from chemotherapy and radiation to Qi Gong and herbal remedies. Hold nothing back because cancer finds weaknesses and exploits them like no other disease."

In the case study first presented in chapter seven, Raymond had quit his Western medical treatment because the medicine was not working and the doctor was now suggesting surgery. I am including it again here, however, to give you an idea of a Qi Gong approach that was used successfully in the treatment of this male cancer.

QI GONG ENERGY TREATMENT

My healing regimen for Raymond began with external Qi treatments, in which I directed Qi to open a number of his meridians, including those governing his liver and kidneys. These were done to improve his energy and blood circulation, both of which would give him a head start in the building of his own internal Qi, which he did through the following exercises.

Three Cancer-Fighting Exercises

To affect his internal Qi, I had Raymond perform the Golden Eight Exercises every day to open his meridians and improve his mental attitude. Through the Golden Eight, we are working the body as a small universe, making sure that all aspects of the body work together in unison. This includes the mental aspects as well. Because Qi Gong exercises call for intense focus, they serve to take the patient's mind off of his cancer, which in turn improves mental attitude. This is important for all patients of chronic illness, since they can suffer from depression as a result of thinking too much about their disease.

"A body that is sick is like a rope tied in knots," I told Raymond. "We use Qi Gong to untie those knots one by one."

I also taught Raymond three new exercises designed specifically for his illness, in addition to the Golden Eight Exercises.

Raymond performed these combined exercises at least two hours a day. This is a lot of time and effort, but it is important, since the Chinese believe that Qi Gong exercises can put you in touch with the healing powers of your subconscious mind.

As I told Raymond, "Once these exercises enter your subconscious mind, they can adjust the health of the body's vital organs."

Each day, when he finished doing the Golden Eight, he did the following three exercises. Through these special techniques of exercise and breathing, we adjust the internal organs and stimulate them with Qi energy and blood.

First Energy Exercise (Figure 12-1)

Sit on the edge of a chair with your body at a ninety-degree angle and with your feet flat on the floor (a). Cross your right leg over your left leg, just above the knee. Grasp your right foot with your left hand in this manner: Place the palm of the hand over the ball of the foot with the fingers firmly grasping the outer edge and the thumb the inner edge. This connects the meridians like a network.

Next, extend your right hand straight out in front of you, with the palm extended upward to release the bad energy (b).

As you inhale, swing your hand to the right as far as possible, keeping your eyes on your hand to receive the proper stretch. At the same time, pull your right foot toward your body with your left hand (c).

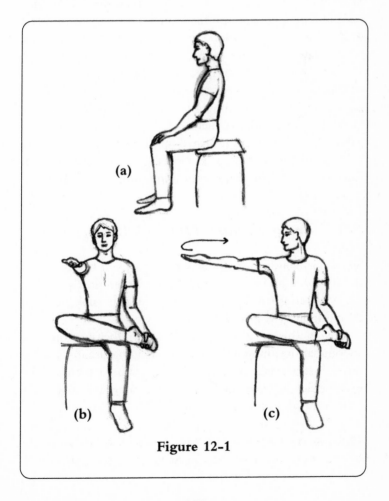

(a)

(b)   **(c)**

Figure 12-1

When you have reached your maximum twist, hold your breath for a moment and then exhale as you return to the starting position.

Repeat this eighteen times on each side.

PURPOSE AND EFFECT: The twist improves circulation along the spine, which in turn stimulates the nerves that reach out to all of the organs. This exercise also opens the liver meridian and directs energy into the kidney and prostate area. The deep breathing forces blood and Qi energy downward into the prostate area, where it contributes to its healing.

Many people who do this exercise actually feel a connection between the kidneys and prostate area, as though there is a charge of energy running between the two areas.

In traditional Chinese medicine, we believe that the open palm in this movement is turned up to the heavens to release bad energy. Think of this palm movement as an object of your focus that helps you divert your mind from your disease.

Second Energy Exercise (Figure 12-2)

Stand normally, feet shoulder-width apart and hands relaxed at your sides (a). Flex your toes upward, then slowly bend at the waist until you are bent over as far as possible, remembering to keep your toes flexed (b).

Stay in this position for one minute, focusing on your abdominal breathing before slowly standing straight. As you do this, stay totally relaxed. Make certain to perform this exercise slowly, since rapid movements can cause back strain.

Perform this two times.

PURPOSE AND EFFECT: In this exercise, the flexion of the toes opens your bladder meridians, which run up the back of your legs, and the kidney meridians found on the inside of the legs. It also circulates energy throughout your body, balancing the yin and yang energy.

On a more mechanical level, this movement forces you to belly breathe, which causes pressure to be put on your intestines and has the effect of massaging the prostate, pushing blood and Qi into the prostate area. In the bent-over position, you will feel the tingling of energy in the lower part of your body and on the backs of your legs. As you stand, the tingling of this energy will move up your back and into your head, opening Qi circulation to the entire body.

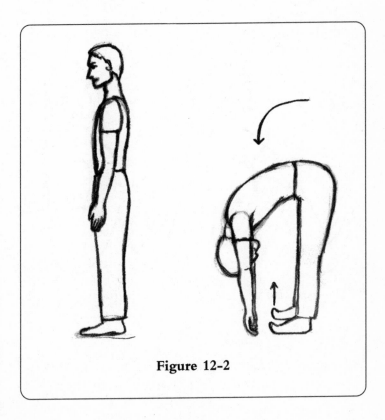

Figure 12-2

Third Energy Exercise (Figure 12-3)

Sit on the floor facing a wall. Place the balls of your feet against a wall and rest your heels on the floor (a). Scoot toward the wall until you are able to wrap your arms around your bent knees. Keeping your back straight, focus on breathing with your stomach, instead of your chest (b).

Breathe in and out eighteen times.

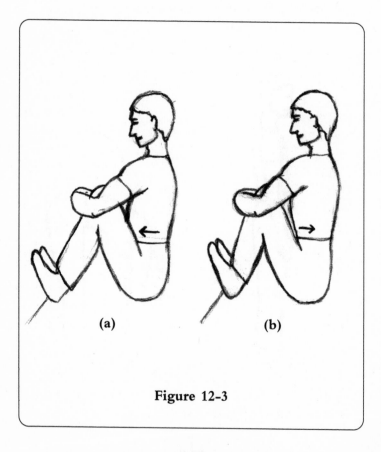

Figure 12-3

PURPOSE AND EFFECT: This exercise focuses energy on the Mei channel that runs through the perineum, which in turn directs energy into the prostate gland. Not only does this exercise put weight on the spine, which stimulates the nerves and improves circulation to the organs, it also forces blood and Qi into the prostate area, while the belly breathing massages the organs. All of these forces combine to force blood and Qi into the area of the prostate gland while massaging it as well.

HERBAL TREATMENTS

There is usually some kind of infection or swelling that precedes prostate cancer, and it is usually a condition that goes on for a long period of time. These are the sort of symptoms that should be recognized and treated. As the ancient physician Wang Ping said, "The superior physician helps before the early budding of the disease." This, of course, is true. But I add to that by saying, "The patient must recognize the early budding of his disease and bring it to the attention of the physician." The following remedies, which I recommended to Raymond, could also help prevent cancer from developing if used in the very earliest stages.

Over a period of three months, Raymond drank the tea from two herbal formulas. These basic formulas focused on the solutions to prostate cancer, including:

- Nourishing the kidney energy and making the spleen healthy
- Promoting pain-free urination
- Increasing the yang energy
- Balancing the energy between the stomach and spleen
- Ridding the body of heat and dampness

Kidney Formula

15 grams	Astragalus root (Huang Qi)
12 grams	Pilose Asiabell root (Dang Shen)
12 grams	Epimedium (Yin Yang Huo)
6 grams	Cistanche (Rou Cong Rong)
6 grams	Morinda root (Ba Ji Tian)
12 grams	Lycium fruit (Gou Qi Zi)
12 grams	Prepared fleeceflower root (He Shou Wu)
15 grams	Anteater scales (Chuan Shan Jia)
12 grams	Cyathula root (Niu Xi)
6 grams	Prepared rhubarb (Da Huang)
10 grams	Prepared philodendron bark (Huang Bai)
6 grams	Anemarrhena rhizome (Zhi Mi)
15 grams	Smilax Glabra rhizome (Tu Fu Ling)
12 grams	Polyphylla Smith (Xi Ye E Zhi Hua)
15 grams	Oldenlandia (Bai Hua She She Cao)
6 grams	Licorice root (Gan Cao)
12 grams	White peony (Bai Shao Yao)

Preparation and prescription: Combine the herbs together in a pot and cover with water, probably about five cups. Boil until they become a thick tea (about three cups' worth) and then pour through a strainer. Drink one glass three times a day for one month.

How it works: This formula is designed to nourish the kidneys by increasing energy flow throughout the body and removing stagnation of the Qi by improving blood circulation and releasing pressure caused by the tumor.

In this formula, astragalus root and pilose asiabell root are combined to improve the circulation throughout the body, increasing the overall Qi level. As the astragalus and pilose increase the overall Qi level of the body, the epimedium, cistanche, morinda root, lycium fruit, fleeceflower root, white peony, and anemarrhena rhizome deliver nutrition directly to the prostate and the kidneys. These herbs help remove infection and swelling (or "heat," as the Chinese refer to it) from the prostate.

Once this heat is removed from the prostate, there are increased levels of toxins in the bloodstream. To help eliminate these extra toxins, six substances are added—cyathula root, rhubarb, philodendron bark, simlax glabra rhizome, and polyphylla Smith—that speed the processing and elimination of toxins.

Anteater scales and cyathula root serve to push the herbal formula downward in the body where it can have the greatest effect upon the prostate problem. (With other illnesses, there are substances added to formulas that push the benefits of the herbal remedy upward.)

Licorice root is added to neutralize toxins that may be present in the herbs themselves.

Oldenlandia is a heat-clearing herb used as a treatment for prostate problems, as well as for sarcoma of the lymph system and carcinomas of the liver and larynx. It is effective with all types of cancer because it increases the production of white blood cells and antibodies. This particular trait also makes it good for the treatment of pneumonia and hepatitis. Because it increases urination and has an antibacterial effect, I have also used it to treat bladder and urinary tract infections.

The herb that has been studied the most in Chinese medicine is astragalus root, which is widely regarded as the king of all herbs. In Chinese medicine, this herb is considered the most powerful because it absorbs the earth's energy best. Modern research tends to agree. Studies done in Japan, China, and the United States show that astragalus alone can lower blood pressure by enlarging blood vessels, reduce blood sugar, and even lessen painful menstrual periods. It has also been found to decrease metabolism and improve heart function.

In China, this herb has been used for hundreds of years to kill tumors. Modern research done in Kyoto Hospital in Japan has confirmed that astragalus can kill many types of cancer cells. In addition, this herb has been found to reduce symptoms associated with the HIV virus by researchers at Lincoln Hospital in New York, where it was given in combination with other herbs to lessen the frequency of night sweats.

Lung and Bladder Formula

6 grams	Ephedra (Ma Huang)
10 grams	Apricot seeds (Xuig Ren)
10 grams	Lepidium (Ting Li)
10 grams	Peucedanum root (Qian Hu)
10 grams	Aster root (Zi Wan)
10 grams	Tussilago flower (Kuan Dong Hua)
10 grams	Ophiopogon root (Mai Men Dong)
15 grams	Chinese lily bulb (Bulbus Lilii) (Bai He)
10 grams	Platycodon root (Jie Geng)
6 grams	Schisandra fruit (Wu Wei Zi)
30 grams	Coix seed (Yi Mi)
10 grams	Alisma tuber (Ze Xie)
20 grams	Poria (Fu Ling)
6 grams	Licorice root (Gan Cao)

Preparation and prescription: Combine the herbs together in a pot and cover with five cups of water. Boil until it becomes a thick tea (about three cups' worth) and then pour through a strainer. Drink one glass three times a day for one month.

How it works: Frequent urination is a problem with prostate cancer patients. It is common for people with this condition to urinate as often as five times per night. This is in part due to a weakening of the muscles that hold urine in our bladders. When these muscles are weakened, they have difficulty holding urine in the bladder and an urgency to urinate is created.

To make the muscles of urination stronger, the formula combines tussilago flower, ophiopogon root, lily bulb, platycodon root, schisandra fruit, coix seed, and alisma tuber. Schisandra has also been shown to have anti-cancer effects. Japanese researchers isolated chemicals in this plant that act as antioxidants, protecting the liver from cancer-causing substances.

Breathing can also be a problem in prostate cancer, since a lack of function in the kidneys often leads to water retention, which makes it difficult to breathe. To improve the function of the lungs, ephedra, apricot seeds, lepidium, peucedanum root, and aster root are combined in this formula. These remedies have long been used by the Chinese to open the lungs' passageways and ease the task of breathing. The apricot seeds contain a substance called isopropylamine, which serves to lower blood pressure, while the remaining ingredients act as diuretics to eliminate excess water from the system.

Another Lung and Bladder Formula

30 grams	Rhubarb (Da Huang)
12 grams	Trichosanthes root (Rian Hua Fen)
12 grams	Mirabilitum (Mang Xiao)
12 grams	Forsythia fruit (Liao Qiao)
9 grams	Immature bitter orange (Zhi Shi)
9 grams	Gardenia fruit (Zhi Zi)
9 grams	Licorice root (Gan Cao)
9 grams	Cotis root (Huang Lian)
24 grams	Radish seed (Lai Fu Zi)
45 grams	Green beans

Preparation and prescription: Combine the herbs together in a pot and cover with five cups of water. Boil until it becomes a thick tea (about three cups' worth) and then pour through a strainer. Drink one glass three times a day for one month.

For serious cases of prostate cancer, I prescribe this same formula as an enema. I have the patients use one-third of this portion three times daily. I have them hold it inside for at least twenty minutes, lying down as they do this to increase the depth that the medication penetrates into the intestines. Not only does this give the body a chance to absorb the herbs, it also relieves constipation, which is a frequent side effect of prostate cancer as well as a source of toxins.

How it works: This formula is designed to detoxify the body by relieving constipation as well as pulling toxins from the bloodstream. This allows the liver to perform its very important job of maintaining blood chemistry without having to filter out the toxins that have built up due to the failure of other systems in the body.

To relieve constipation and clean the large intestine, I have combined rhubarb, trichosanthes root, mirabilitum, forsythia fruit, and cotis root. These substances are frequently used in Chinese medicine to clean the large intestine, which is the longest and largest internal organ in the body. Rhubarb functions as a bulk laxative that, when combined with the purgative effects of the other herbs, serves to clear the large intestine.

As a means of clearing toxins from the blood and encouraging Qi and blood flow through the liver meridian, I have combined immature bitter orange, gardenia fruit, radish seed, and green beans. These have long been used in Chinese medicine as a means of detoxifying the liver. Even in Western medicine, substances like green beans have been recommended as a means of pulling cholesterol from the bloodstream, which is a toxin of sorts to healthy arteries. One of the most active of these herbs is the bitter orange. Not only does it stimulate the liver and gallbladder, it also contains phenolic acid, which makes it an anti-inflammatory.

Finally I have included licorice root, which I call the king of herbs. Not only does this common herb add flavor, it also neutralizes many toxins.

That is the reason I recommend licorice tea to many of my cancer patients. I have them drop twigs of this root into hot water and drink two cups of the tea per day.

Whenever Raymond's condition changed, I varied the formula. For instance, when he had extreme difficulty with urination I added aquilaria wood (Chen Xiang), cucuma root (Yu Jin), and kindera root (Wu Yao)—all herbs that help relax the muscles of the urethra. Sometimes for painful urination I would add corydalis tuber (Yan Hu Sao), vaccaria seed (Wang Bu Lix Xing), bureed tuber (San Leng), and redoary (E Zhu); this herbal combination has a painkilling effect upon the urinary system.

To reduce swelling in the prostate I would sometimes add Japanese thistle (Xiao Ji), eclipta (Han Liau Cao), rehmannia root (Sheng di), and donkey hide gelatin (E Jiao) to the above formula. In addition to the reduced swelling and analgesic effect, these herbs energize the kidneys and help draw infection from the body.

An interesting note: At one point during my treatment of Raymond he had blood in his urine and a painful bladder. I prescribed sixteen ounces of goat's milk, which he was to drink daily for days. This simple remedy relieved his problem.

FOODS THAT FIGHT CANCER

There are specific foods and dietary guidelines that will treat cancer of specific organs. Some of these dietary recommendations have healing properties, while all of them make it easier for the specific organ to function.

Prostate Cancer. Foods of the sea are the most effective ones for prostate cancer. These include seaweed (soaked in water first to remove the salt), seaweed tea (which is about ten ounces of seaweed boiled in water for two minutes), and mussels. Other healing foods include bamboo shoots and garlic, which can be cooked and eaten with steamed vegetables.

Stomach Cancer. Because this type of cancer usually results in indigestion, it is advised that you avoid spicy foods as well as stimulants like coffee and tea. It is also advisable to avoid liquor and tobacco, since they irritate the lining of the stomach. To help soothe the stomach, eat foods like corn, mushrooms, bean sprouts, spinach, and rice milk, all of which are easy to digest.

A natural remedy to help control the spread of cancer is sunflower stems. About four ounces of dried stems boiled in a pan of water (approximately one quart) for about two minutes can be sipped daily as a means of slowing the growth of the disease. I recommend drinking two cups per day.

Lung Cancer. This is an extremely uncomfortable disease that carries such symptoms as coughing, shortness of breath, and even the expectoration of bloody mucus. To fight these symptoms, I recommend the consumption of almonds, spinach, jellyfish, lotus seeds and roots, pears, Chinese white tree bark fungus (Yin Er), and soybean milk. Moderate amounts of these foods will help remedy these conditions.

Liver Cancer. Since one of the roles of the liver is to help in the digestion of food, persons with liver cancer should eat only moderately. They should consume foods that are easy to digest. There are many foods in this category, including green beans, fruits, pheasant eggs, and garlic. When fluid retention occurs in the stomach and the abdomen is swollen, corn, red beans, winter melon, and fish soup with onion are recommended.

Intestinal and Colon Cancer. One of the main symptoms of this type of cancer is diarrhea and bloody stools. Foods that can improve bowel movements are figs, green beans, celery, bananas, pears, seaweed, and honey.

Breast Cancer. I recommend a diet of clams and crab for breast cancer, as well as bamboo shoots and lichee nuts.

Although food is not thought of as medicine by Western doctors, it is hard to ignore its healing properties. The recommendations I've just given provide the extra energy and nutrients that the system needs to help it fight illness.

The following recipe is one that I recommended to Raymond to help fight his prostate cancer.

Medicinal Lamb with Herbs

1 ounce	Dioscorea (Shan Yao)
½ ounce	Lindera Root (Wu Yao)
½ ounce	Black Cardamom Seed (Yi Zhi Ren)
½ ounce	Ginger, sliced
1 ounce	Scallions
½ cup	Rice wine
1 teaspoon	Salt
¼ teaspoon	White pepper
1	Egg white
16 ounces	Chicken broth
1 tablespoon	Cornstarch
1 bunch	Spinach
1 pound	Lamb kidney

Preparation and prescription: Combine the herbs in a pot with two cups of water. Bring to a boil, then turn the heat down and simmer until it has boiled down to one-quarter cup. Set aside.

Slice the lamb kidneys lengthwise and remove the vines. Slice into six pieces and wash them with water, then press them dry. Combine pieces in a bowl with the wine, ginger, scallions, salt, egg white, and cornstarch. Set aside.

Wash the spinach and cook it in boiling water for thirty seconds. Drain.

Take the herbs out of the pot, keeping the juice inside. Add chicken broth to the herb broth and bring to a boil. Add the lamb slices and cook until they are tender. Add the white pepper, salt to taste, spinach, and serve.

How it works: This medicinal dish adds heat to the kidneys, which are made cold by the cancer, according to Chinese medicine. The added heat not only improves the function of the kidneys, it also takes the pain out of urination. Much of the medicinal effect is due to the herbs that are used. The dioscorea, for instance, stimulates the function of the stomach and spleen, while the lindera root and the black cardamom seed warm the kidneys and improve their function.

The Chinese myth about dioscorea (Shan Yao) deals with its ability to renew strength. It goes like this:

In ancient China, a tribe of farmers was attacked by a savage tribe and driven from their land. The attackers drove the farmers into the mountains, where they were left to die by the savages, who thought there was no food. The farmers were indeed in trouble, until they found a meadow filled with a white flowering plant. Out of desperation, they ate the roots and became stronger and stronger by the day. Finally they banded together and attacked the savages. A brutal fight ensued and all of the savages were either killed or driven from their land.

The farmers continued to eat the roots, which they named Shan (mountain) Yao (earth) and were never attacked again.

Whether or not this myth is true, it is most certainly an apt metaphor for the energy-building properties of this sweet root and its ability to drive disease from the body.

It is easy to see how my treatment can fit in with Western methods of treating prostate cancer. Just be sure to discuss other treatments with your doctor. I cannot emphasize enough my belief that the battle against cancer should include the best that both Eastern and Western medicine have to offer. Said an ancient philosopher, "The wise man knows that he should not lift something heavy with one hand when two hands are available."

13

Headaches

According to Hua Tuo, a noted physician of ancient China, "Dislike of work is just as important [a factor in illness] as not taking care of one's body."

Although this statement is two thousand years old, it is a very contemporary viewpoint. Many people are affected by their jobs. Although they may not dislike what they do, they certainly feel the pressures of their careers. Many times, these stresses manifest themselves in the form of headaches.

A prime example of this was a patient I had in Shanghai, a mid-level bureaucrat who was the victim of a daily headache. He said headaches hit him every afternoon shortly after lunch. He would be sitting at his desk, performing the boring task of compiling statistics from some kind of official record book, when he would be struck by sharp pains in his head.

"Sometimes it feels as though a worm is in my brain," he said. "The pain is terrible and it only stops if I lean back and think about my job and nothing else."

I was puzzled by that comment, since thinking about work is a frequent cause of headaches and not a cure. I asked him about his diet, and whether he was drinking much more tea than usual.

"I do not overeat and I certainly do not drink too much tea," he insisted.

"Is your job stressful?" I asked.

"No, but it is a job that I hate," he said. "If my father had not gotten me this job I would never work here. But now that I have taken the job, I have to keep it. If I didn't, my father would be embarrassed by my quitting."

I was puzzled. "I thought your headache went away when you thought about your job," I said. "To me that seems as though you must like it."

The young man sighed. "It doesn't work that way with me," he said. "When I get the headache I am daydreaming about what it is I really want to do, which is to become an artist. I imagine myself in a beautiful place painting the scenery around me and I get a terrible headache. It is only by blocking out those thoughts and focusing on where I really am that my headache goes away."

I felt sorry for the young man because he did not have the freedom to do what he wanted. Still, my job was that of physician and I did what I was supposed to do, which was diagnose his problem and offer him some remedy. After a number of questions that eliminated organic problems, I decided that what he suffered from were simple headaches.

In Chinese medicine, the excessive presence of Yang energy, along with the accumulation of bad energy, causes a blockage of energy in the head. When this blockage occurs, energy cannot circulate as freely as it would in a healthy person; the excess cannot be lowered from the head and the problem cannot be rectified. This cause can be further categorized as two types: the simple headache—Xie Qi in Chinese—caused by intermittent blockages that affect nerves in the brain; and the complex or chronic headache—Yuan Qi—which is caused by prolonged blockages, where the blood vessels are adversely affected and the person experiences pain continuously.

Aside from the aforementioned, headaches may also be caused by physical trauma to the head.

Western medicine divides headaches into two basic categories as well. The migraine headache is caused by the blood vessels of the brain constricting and then dilating. This uneven flow of blood leads to vision disturbances, severe pain, and sometimes even nausea.

The second type is the tension headache. Tension or stress constricts the blood vessels to the brain, generally resulting in throbbing pain in all or part of the head. It can be caused by any number of things, including stress, eye strain, poor diet, alcohol, allergies, and menstrual cycles.

For both types of headaches, Western physicians recommend pain relievers like aspirin or acetaminophen, changes in diet, or even stress-reduction training. Some of the more heavy-duty approaches to treatment include antihistamines to expand blood vessels, vasoconstrictors to narrow blood vessels, or beta blockers to keep blood vessels from constricting or dilating.

In Chinese medicine, both types of headaches, simple or constant, require exercises to open the blocked meridian channels. For the simple headache, the goal is to take energy that has collected in the head and bring it down into the body. For the constant headache, the goal is to adjust the internal organs of the body by opening their meridian channels. With both types, however, the focus can be to move bad energy out of the head.

The following exercises are aimed at doing just that. Before doing these exercises, you can practice the Golden Eight exercises. They do open meridian channels, which will usually provide relief. If they do not work, or if you simply want to try something different, here are two more possibilities. I prescribed these exercises to the young man who had a headache every afternoon at work. He did them every day shortly after lunch. He still daydreamed, yet he no longer had his headaches. In America I learned that this is known as "having your cake and eating it, too."

Had the exercises alone not eliminated his headaches, I would have prescribed the herbal remedy that follows for simple headache. Since the exercises alone were sufficient, I let well enough alone in his case.

Exercise for Clearing Your Head (Figure 13-1)

Sitting cross-legged on the floor, focus on your perineum, the area just below your rectum. As you inhale, contract this muscle and imagine that you are bringing the energy of this contraction up through the body to the top of your head. Then, as you exhale, relax your perineum and imagine bringing the energy from your head back down through your body.

Concentrate on your breathing and also on the flexing and relaxing of your perineum.

Do this approximately thirty times and then open your eyes and relax. If your headache persists, repeat another thirty times.

PURPOSE AND EFFECT: There are a number of special meridian channels in Chinese medicine, but the most important are the governing vessel meridian and the conception vessel meridian. The governing meridian runs down your back from the top of the head to the perineum, where it joins the conception meridian, which runs up the front of your body to your chin. The governing meridian controls the Qi of all of the yang meridians, while the conception meridian controls the yin meridians. By unblocking both meridians, this exercise balances the yin and yang energy that is out of balance in your head.

In Western terms, this exercise relaxes the neck, spine, and legs, and slows your heartbeat and allows your blood vessels to relax.

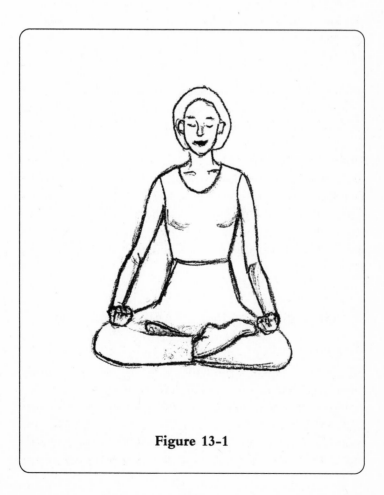

Figure 13-1

Foot Meditation

Another simple yet effective exercise is to focus on the Yong Quan point, which is located on the bottom of the foot in the middle of the arch. This Qi spot is on the left foot for men and the right foot for women, and connects to every organ in the body.

Sitting cross-legged on the floor (as in Figure 13-1), let the foot with the Yong Quan point be on top. Then concentrate, focusing your energy on that point. Do this for approximately ten to twenty minutes and see how you feel. If you do not feel better, then apply pressure to the Yong Quan point with your thumb for about five minutes, moving your thumb fifty-four times in a counterclockwise direction and fifty-four times in a clockwise direction.

PURPOSE AND EFFECT: It may seem odd to a Western reader that the treatment for a headache involves treating the feet. But in Chinese medicine, a different area is often treated to pull bad energy away from the afflicted area. In this case, concentrating on the Yong Quan point, and even applying pressure with your finger if needed, pulls the extra Qi from your head.

HERBS FOR SIMPLE AND COMPLEX HEADACHES

"If you are thinking good thoughts," an old saying goes, "your head will feel the pleasant effects of good energy."

Unfortunately, it is not always the good energy of life that finds its way to the head. Sometimes there are causes for headaches that you have no control over, like a bad environment. And sometimes there are thoughts that you cannot control that make you tense and fill your head with bad Qi. There are hundreds of causes of headaches, and Chinese medicine has dozens of remedies for each category of headache. I provide my two favorites here.

There are generally three ways to take Chinese medicine. The most popular way is in a decoction, which is the way most of the formulas in this book are presented. Another way is to combine herbs with something like honey and roll them up into pills. The third is to crush the herbs into a powder. The first remedy included here is taken in a powder form. Not only is it extremely effective in this way, but it is also easily carried with you. This remedy is so effective for simple headaches that it is common to see people in China carrying small amounts of it in snuff boxes.

Remedy for a Simple Headache

9 grams	Cnidium (Chuan Xiang)
9 grams	Mastic (Ru Xiang)
9 grams	Myrrh (Mo Yao)
9 grams	Polygala root (Yuan Zhi)
9 grams	Asarum (Xi Xin)
9 grams	Gypsum (Shi Gao)
9 grams	Trichosanthes root (Rian Hua Fen)

Preparation and prescription: Combine all of the herbs and grind them into a fine powder with a mortar and pestle. If the left side of your head hurts, sniff a small amount of this powder into your right nostril. If the right side of your head hurts, sniff it up your left nostril. If both sides hurt, put it up both nostrils.

Do this no more than three times per day.

How it works: This formula is especially effective for people who are constantly on the run and have very tense jobs. I sometimes call these "high-tech" headaches because people who work around computers and other sorts of technology that pressure them all day are usually the ones who suffer from this malady.

I have combined cnidium, mastic, and myrrh and polygala root to enhance the circulation of blood and energy to the brain. Asarum and gypsum are combined to help the medicine penetrate where it is needed, while trichosanthes root is added to pull out the bad energy.

Western medical research backs up the traditional Chinese view of these herbs. Although myrrh was used in the embalming process by the ancient Egyptians and is now used as an antiseptic in mouthwash, recent research has shown that it contains chemicals that stimulate the circulation, which is the reason it works so well as an herb used in headache relief. This is especially true when myrrh is combined with mastic, a form of resin from the mastic tree. Although a source of incense and perfume, mastic is also known to stop pain and swelling, and achieves especially deep penetration when combined with the circulation-stimulating effects of myrrh.

Remedy for a Constant Headache

9 grams	Bupleurum root (Chai Hu)
10 grams	Red peony (Zi Bai Shao)
10 grams	White peony (Bai Shao)
10 grams	Cyperus tuber (Xiang Fu)
10 grams	Citrus leaf (Jie Yei)
9 grams	Bitter orange
6 grams	Licorice root (Gan Cao)

Preparation and prescription: Combine all of the herbs together in a pot and add filtered water until they are covered. Boil this mixture until about one-third of the water is gone. Strain the herbs from the thick tea and store in a jar or pitcher.

Drink one cup of this decoction in the morning and a second cup in the afternoon. If you need to, drink a third cup after dinner. To prevent stomachache, however, always drink this tea after meals.

Purpose and effect: In traditional Chinese medicine, we say that the pressures of life can become so great that they force bad energy out of the liver and into the head. To counteract this, I combined bupleurum root, red peony, white peony, and cyperus tuber. These help open the liver meridian so good energy can flow. The cyperus tuber also acts with the citrus leaf and bitter orange to get rid of the toxins in the blood.

Some of the most recent research to arouse the interest of international drug companies was conducted with bupleurum root. In Chinese medicine, this root is used to clear toxins from the blood as well as to clean the blood of bacteria and viruses. Japanese medical researchers at Osaka's City General Hospital decided to study the Chinese claims for this herb and found that cirrhosis patients who took the herb had better liver function and therefore a lower incidence of liver cancer and a longer rate of survival than other patients who did not take the herb. This is important when considering headaches, since we believe that many headaches are caused by blockage of the liver meridian.

FOODS FOR HEADACHE RELIEF

I always ask dietary questions of anyone who comes to me with a headache. Even though food might not be the cause of a headache, it can certainly make a headache worse. People who drink a lot of caffeine or eat a lot of chocolate, or who have stopped consuming these products, are sometimes as subject to headaches as those who have stressful jobs.

But just as food can sometimes lead to headache, it can also be used to get rid of a headache. Simple foods like bananas and other fruits can help a headache go away. There are also more exciting dishes that have curative effects on headaches, like the one that follows.

Sautéed Diced Fish

½ ounce	Gastrodia tuber (Tian Ma)
½ ounce	Cnidium (Chuan Xiang)
1 ounce	Lycium fruit (Gou Qi Zi)
1½ pounds	White fish, diced
1	Green pepper, sliced
1	Egg white
½ tablespoon	White pepper
1 tablespoon	Cooking wine
1 tablespoon	Scallion, diced
1 tablespoon	Ginger
½ teaspoon	Honey
2 tablespoons	Cornstarch, divided
¼ cup	Chicken broth
6 tablespoons	Sesame oil, divided

Preparation and prescription: Combine the fish in a bowl with honey, white pepper, egg white, the juice made from the boiled herbs, one tablespoon of sesame oil, and one tablespoon of cornstarch.

Add four tablespoons of sesame oil to a skillet and add the fish mixture to the skillet while the oil is still cold. Cook until the fish is about half done and then set it aside.

Sauté scallions, green pepper, ginger, and lycium fruit in one tablespoon of sesame oil. Add the cooking wine and chicken broth and bring to a boil. Then add the fish and cook until it is done.

In a cup combine the remaining cornstarch with water to make a paste. Add this paste to the mixture and serve immediately.

How it works: Cnidium counteracts the excess of energy in the head that causes headaches, by improving blood circulation, and works as a general pain reliever. Cnidium and gastrodia tuber combine to quell a hyperactive liver, or, as we say, remove some of the yang.

Granted, headaches sometimes spring up with no apparent cause. But if you are having frequent headaches, it might be best to deal with the true source. The ultimate cure for a headache may not lie in medicine, but in lifestyle.

14

Hypertension

Hypertension and job stress go hand in hand. At the credit-checking company TRW, for instance, I was asked to conduct an eight-week clinic on stress reduction. The company had been having problems with complaints of high stress among its employees and wanted to see what effect, if any, Qi Gong would have on the reduction of stress in the workforce.

Since the manager who hired me wanted an objective measure of stress reduction, I decided to measure changes in blood pressure. Because stress is one of the causes of high blood pressure, I reasoned that if stress decreased, so would blood pressure.

High blood pressure causes the blood vessels to constrict and increase the pressure required to pump blood through them. When this happens, heart attacks, strokes, and kidney damage become much more likely. High blood pressure is a major concern in the West. When a person is diagnosed with high blood pressure, he or she is likely to be put on one of a variety of antihypertensive medications. These drugs reduce blood pressure in a number of ways. Diuretics, for instance, increase the speed with which your body eliminates salt and urine. This in turn decreases the pressure within your blood vessels. A side effect of diuretics is the increased loss of potassium, which may cause irregular heartbeat. Beta blockers may also be prescribed. These prevent small arteries from becoming smaller and increasing blood pressure. Some physicians are concerned about the use of these drugs because there is evidence that they may increase the chance of heart attacks.

I understand that a drug approach may sometimes be necessary. In my experience, however, I have found very few cases of hypertension that do not respond to Qi Gong exercises. If the exercises alone do not work, I will then recommend changes in lifestyle to go along with them. It is the rare case of high blood pressure that does not respond to weight loss. Even the loss of a few pounds can lead to substantial changes in blood pressure readings. The same is true of cigarette smoking and heavy alcohol consumption; when those are stopped or even curtailed, blood pressure will certainly drop.

To the Chinese way of thinking, there would be no reason to give drugs for hypertension before making changes in lifestyle. To do that would be to treat the symptom and not the cause of the disease. Generally I would prescribe exercises to open the kidney meridians. By opening the kidney meridian, we calm the patient by cleaning the blood of such elements as adrenaline. This also has the effect of lowering the cholesterol levels in the blood.

I had my hypertension patients at TRW follow a three-step process of exercises. These are progressive exercises, which means the patients did not go on to the next one until they had reached the specific goal of the exercise they were doing. These patients did the Golden Eight in addition to the exercises described here. By diligently following the exercise prescription, they were able to reach their goal to:

- Lower blood pressure
- Stabilize blood pressure
- Provide deep relaxation and get the mind off the source of their stress

By the end of the clinic, the average systolic blood pressure (the heart contracting) reading dropped twenty-three points and the average diastolic (the heart relaxed) dropped eleven points. These results came about without any medications or herbal remedies. My only tool in lowering their blood pressure was teaching my students to control the flow of their Qi. The body's goal is to maintain health. With a disease like hypertension, a patient can easily realize this goal through focus, breath, and form.

Step One: Vision Shower (Figure 14-1)

Stand relaxed, feet shoulder-width apart and your knees slightly bent (a). Raise your arms with elbows turned slightly outward to keep your armpits open (b). Hands are at waist level with palms pointed toward the ground and relaxed, as if pressing lightly on a balloon. Your thumbs and forefingers should be level with an area about one inch below your navel. This area is referred to as the *dan tien*.

Inhale deeply through your nose, contracting your anus to pull Qi to the lower part of your body and slowly raising your hands to the middle of your chest; then exhale as you relax your anus and lower your hands to the *dan tien*. As you inhale, keep the tip of your tongue on the roof of your mouth. As you exhale, let it relax to a normal position. Breathe eight to ten times per minute.

As you breathe, visualize warm water running down your body from your head to your feet. Keep your eyes slightly opened and focused on the tip of your nose.

Do this exercise in a quiet place with good air circulation for twenty minutes, one or two times per day. This is not a vigorous exercise. Rather, it is a peaceful meditation, so direct your mind accordingly.

PURPOSE AND EFFECT: This exercise provides the kind of relaxation that leads to lower blood pressure, probably because it slows respiration and heart rate and leads to the

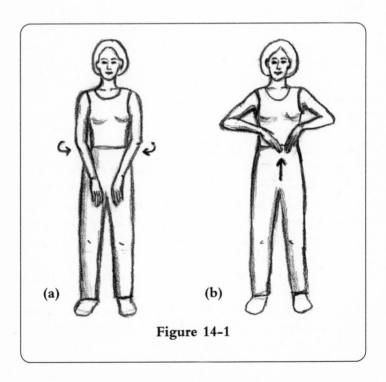

Figure 14-1

relaxation of tense arteries. Your blood pressure should drop significantly, perhaps twenty systolic points and ten diastolic points within ten days of doing this exercise.

Step Two: First Exercise to Stabilize Blood Pressure (Figure 14-2)

Do not do this exercise until your blood pressure is lowered from Step One.

Sit on the front third of a chair, with your spine erect and your body relaxed (Figure 14-2). With your palms facing each other and your forearms parallel to the ground, hold

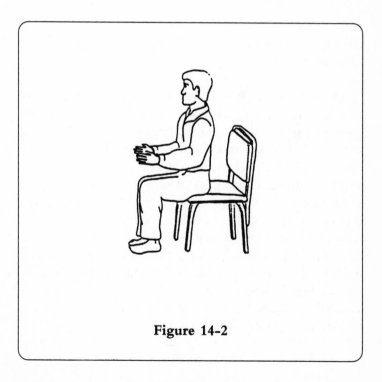

Figure 14-2

your arms approximately a foot apart. Keep your hands stationary as you breathe deeply and slowly, approximately eight to ten times per minute. As you do this, visualize a balloon between your hands as you concentrate on your lower *dan tien*, that spot about one inch below your navel.

Your rate of breathing should be about eight to ten breaths a minute for about thirty minutes. Perform this exercise twice daily, morning and evening.

PURPOSE AND EFFECT: This exercise leads to further physical relaxation, while improving the mental ability to relax, as well. This is done through visualization techniques that help you direct your Qi to the lower part of your body, where it is no longer a source of high blood pressure.

Second Exercise to Stabilize Blood Pressure (Figure 14-3)

Using the standing form in Step One with your hands parallel to your sides, visualize your hands floating on water. Note that your thumbs and forefingers are level with your *dan tien*. Relax your total body, with specific emphasis on relaxing your lower abdomen, shoulders, and elbows. Smile slightly with mouth and lips closed.

Breathe as directed in Step One, at a rate of eight to ten times per minute, without moving your arms.

Focus on your feet as they become hot and tingly. As you focus on them, you will notice that they tingle more and become hotter with each breath. You will also have the feeling that they are expanding.

Do this exercise for about ten minutes and repeat it three to four times per day, for fifteen days.

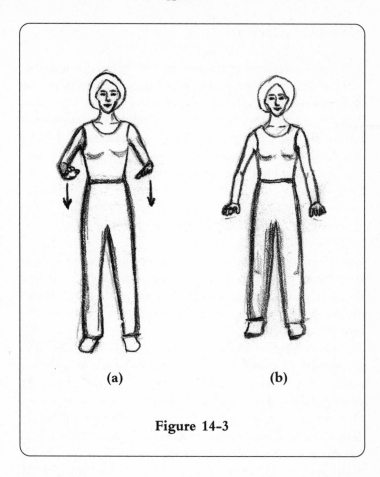

(a)   (b)

Figure 14-3

PURPOSE AND EFFECT: As you perform this exercise, Qi and blood will move from your head to the lower parts of your body. This should lower and stabilize your blood pressure, especially when you are standing. This exercise successfully lowers the blood pressure in about eighty-five percent of the patients who practice it for at least three months.

Maintenance Exercises

The following three exercises are similar to meditations. After your blood pressure has been reduced using steps one and two, you can perform these exercises to maintain your lower blood pressure. Many patients find the one in particular that they like and perform that one periodically. Others will do all three or mix and match. It does not matter which one you do, as long as it works for you.

Exercise to Lower Blood Pressure (Figure 14-4)

Use the same form as illustrated in Step One, except allow your hands to remain relaxed at your sides. With your feet shoulder-width apart, your chin lowered, and your eyes and mouth slightly opened, place the tip of your tongue on the roof of your mouth.

Press on your navel forty-nine times at a rate of one time per second. Men should use the middle finger of their left hand, and women the middle finger of their right hand. As you inhale and press on this acupressure point, visualize the Qi moving up from the balls of your feet through the inside of your legs and into the lower *dan tien*. As you exhale, imagine warm water running down your body from your head, across your neck and shoulders, and down to your feet. As the water flows over each part of your body, tell those parts to relax.

Do this exercise for at least fifteen minutes and no more than one hour.

Finish this relaxing exercise by briskly rubbing your hands together until they are hot, and then massage your face sixteen times with the palms of your hands.

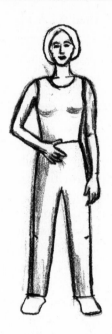

Figure 14-4

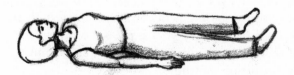

Figure 14-5

PURPOSE AND EFFECT: Do not eat too much before doing this exercise. If you are tired, lie down and perform the exercise. This is an especially good exercise if you are having trouble sleeping.

Visualization Exercise (Figure 14-5)

Lie flat on the bed or floor and completely relax your body. Close your eyes and breathe normally and keep your arms at your sides with both palms either up or down. Then repeat the following procedure:

Close your eyes for two seconds and then open for two seconds. Repeat three times. Then open your eyes and look up toward the top of your head. Keep your eyes open for two seconds, then close them for two seconds. Then look down toward your feet. Bring your eyes back to center, look left and then right. In each position, open your eyes for two seconds and then close for two seconds. Repeat these movements two to three times.

Open your mouth wide and gently curl your tongue to the back of the roof of your mouth. Close your mouth, keeping your tongue in that position. Hold to a count of ten before opening your mouth and releasing your tongue to its normal position. Repeat this movement three times.

Close your eyes and concentrate on your toes. Relax your body in stages, starting with your toes, then feet, then ankles, calves, and continue up your body. Relax your body in sections all the way to the top of your head. Completely relax each part before moving on.

Visualize a quiet and beautiful place. Imagine yourself there, breathing in the clean fresh air. Take as much energy from this special place as it can give you. As you do this, breathe from your lower abdomen slowly and deeply, ten to twelve times.

When you finish, you will feel deeply relaxed. Savor the feeling for several seconds and then slowly sit up and stretch.

Do this once a day for ten minutes.

PURPOSE AND EFFECT: In the same way that visualizing a tense scene can cause your muscles to contract, visualizing a calming one can cause your muscles to relax. This is the body's relaxation response and includes involuntary muscles like the heart and the arteries.

Ankle Roll (Figure 14-6)

Sitting on a chair, rest one ankle on the opposite knee. Hold your toes in one hand and support your ankle with the other. Slowly rotate your foot and ankle thirty to forty times each way for each foot.

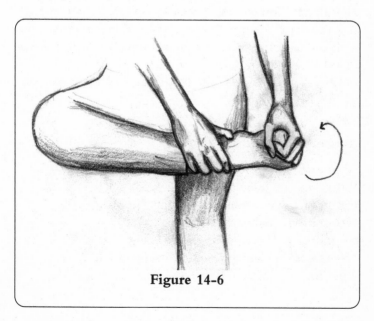

Figure 14-6

Do this once in the morning and once in the evening with each foot.

PURPOSE AND EFFECT: According to the practice of Qi Gong, people with very still ankles and toes will have high blood pressure. This is because your feet have the most pressure points of any part of the body and are also the beginning and ending points of the meridians. Rotating the feet in this manner moves Qi through your meridians, which will have a positive effect on all other parts of the body.

HERBS FOR HYPERTENSION

As I pointed out earlier, hypertension can usually be controlled through exercise alone. That is usually the best option, since hypertension drugs have many undesirable side effects. Sometimes, however, exercise is not enough and you have to turn to medication. When that happens with my patients, I make an herbal powder called Apricot Blood Pressure Powder.

Overall, this is one of the best formulas I know for controlling hypertension.

Apricot Blood Pressure Powder

90 grams	Apricot seed (Xing Ren)
150 grams	Tribulus fruit (Ci Ji Li)
150 grams	Scrophularia (Xuan Sheu)
150 grams	Salvia (Dan Shen)
60 grams	Areca seed (Bing Lang)
150 grams	Plantago seed (Che Qian Zi)
9 grams	Amber (Hu Po)

Preparation and prescription: Combine the ingredients and grind them into a powder. Drink five grams of the powder mixed with fruit juice twice a day, in the morning and the evening.

How it works: The herbs in this powder are aimed at clearing the kidney meridian, which is seen in Chinese medicine as the main cause of high blood pressure. The way we view it, the lung is metal and the kidney is wood. In this case, that means that we use the power of the lung to chop away the weaknesses of the kidney. To build the strength of the lungs, I have used apricot seed, which is one of the most effective herbs for improving the function of the lungs and the liver.

To clear such elements as adrenaline from the bloodstream, I add tribulus fruit, scrophularia, and salvia. These substances are known to clear the blood of toxins. Salvia in particular is a well-known antibacterial agent that has long been used as a means of stopping sweating and drying up the flow of breast milk.

Areca seed and plantago seed are added as a diuretic to get rid of excess water that makes it harder for the heart to pump blood. Plantago seed, by the way, is best known in the West as psyllium, which is used as a bulk laxative as well as a way of lowering blood cholesterol levels. Amber is added to direct the medicine's energy downward.

BLOOD PRESSURE BATTLERS

It is impossible to ignore the role that diet plays in raising and lowering blood pressure. Even Confucius acknowledged the damage that diet can cause to the Qi when he said, "If one is too full, it robs him of vitality and spirit as well as causing shortness of breath."

Like many Western doctors, I think a key to improving one's dietary health lies in eating a breakfast that is not only fat-free, but actually serves to clean the blood of cholesterol and fat. I call such a meal a "medicinal breakfast," and often recommend the following dish to anyone who is serious about healing his hypertension.

Healing Rice

1 cup	Black rice (available at Chinese markets)
1 cup	Chinese red beans, dried
1 cup	Lotus seeds
1 cup	Dried Chestnuts

Preparation and prescription: Soak the ingredients overnight in separate containers.

Combine the rice and beans in a covered pot with four cups of water and bring them to a boil. Then reduce heat and simmer for one and a half hours.

In another covered pot, combine the lotus seeds with four cups of water and bring to a boil for fifteen minutes. Then reduce to medium heat for forty-five minutes or until the seeds are soft.

In a third covered pot, boil the water chestnuts for five minutes and then pour the water off to eliminate the bitter taste. Then add four cups of fresh water and bring to a boil. Then turn the fire down to a medium heat and let them simmer for twenty minutes.

Combine the lotus seeds and their juice to the rice and beans. Drain the water chestnuts and add them to the beans, rice, and lotus seeds.

Add honey, sugar, or sweetener to taste and you have a wonderful medicinal meal.

How it works: There is nothing magical about this dish except its taste. It is a high-fiber, low-fat meal that absorbs cholesterol from the body. Its effect is similar to that of oatmeal, but its taste is far more interesting.

Chicken Soup

1 ounce	Lycium fruit (Gou Qi Zi)
½ ounce	Pseudo ginseng (San Qi)
½ ounce	Eucommia bark (Du Zhong)
1	Whole chicken
1 bunch	Scallions, cut 1 inch long
30 grams	Ginger
½ cup	Rice wine
2 teaspoons	Salt
6 cups	Water

Preparation and prescription: Wash whole chicken and stuff with pseudo ginseng and eucommia bark.

Put the chicken into a pot with all the other ingredients and cover with six cups or more of water. Bring contents of the pot to a boil and then simmer for three hours. Shred chicken meat into broth for soup, or drink the broth plain.

How it works: In many cultures, chicken soup is recommended as a cure-all, especially for colds, headaches, or even just bad days. The Chinese also recommend chicken soup for ailments. In this case the chicken soup has herbal ingredients that act to lower high blood pressure. Pseudo ginseng is a known anti-inflammatory that also acts to lower blood pressure. The eucommia bark stimulates liver and kidney function and, among other things, serves as a diuretic to get rid of excess water in the body, which can cause high blood pressure.

★ ★ ★

Hypertension is one of the most common diseases in the Western world. It is also one of the easiest problems to eliminate. Usually the only thing required is diet and exercise and sometimes stress reduction. As a physician who believes in a holistic approach, I always insist that my hypertension patients try a nonmedicinal approach to this problem. It is only if that approach fails that I move on to the herbal remedies.

"If the atmosphere of Yang is exposed to great anger," reads *The Yellow Emperor's Classic of Internal Medicine*, "the force of life of the body is interrupted and the blood rushes upwards and causes dizziness."

Fortunately, we know the simple steps that can bring the Qi back into balance.

15

Stress and Depression

Stress and depression are like two frightened sisters, say the Chinese, because they often go hand in hand. I have seen the truth of this statement many times. We all face stress and depression sometime in our lives. Whether it is sickness and death or family and business problems, unhappiness waits around the corner for us all.

Sometimes it seems to all strike at once. Such was the case with a colleague of mine, a medical doctor whom I will call Thomas. He was a well-respected doctor who owned his own clinic in the Los Angeles area. A graduate of a major California medical school, he was tall, athletic, and hand-some, with a wonderful temperament and a patient-pleasing bedside manner. Since his family was wealthy, he had never experienced financial hardships. He had a beautiful wife and two children, a son and daughter. Life had been good to him.

All of that suddenly changed. He called one day and asked if he could come by for a consultation. I had not seen him in at least two years, so I was not prepared for the change I saw. When he got out of his car I could see that he was in terrible shape both mentally and physically. His body was bent, as though something horrible had drained it of energy. His face and eyes were puffy and red. It was clear from the way he carried himself that something very emotional was pressuring his chest.

I scanned him in the treatment room to see what else was wrong with him. Using my Qi Gong perception, I could see that much bad energy had collected in his liver and filled it up. His lungs were congested with phlegm and all of his internal organs seemed completely unbalanced. He told me that he could not eat, and when he lay down, he could not sleep. To make matters worse, he had to urinate frequently during the night.

Through simple observation I could see that Thomas's life had somehow taken a terrible turn. Because of it, he was in extreme distress. I told him a story that would help him put his thoughts in order.

When I was in China, I traveled a lot because I wanted to collect all of the different energies found in various parts of the country. One place I visited was Yunnan. This is a beautiful tropical province in south China where people have the particularly disgusting (to outsiders, at least) habit of hunting monkeys so they can eat their brains.

One of the hunters I spoke to told of a time when he captured a baby monkey. Just as he was about to put it in a cage, he saw the mother watching him from the jungle. He wanted the mother, since she was larger and would fetch more money on the market. He decided to kill the baby, thinking that the mother would approach in hopes of saving her child. He pulled a knife and began to cut the baby open before the mother's eyes. The mother began to go berserk. She jumped up and down and screamed at the horror she was forced to witness. Then she simply fell to earth and died.

The hunter wondered what had happened to kill the mother. He examined the dead mother monkey and could see nothing wrong on the outside. Still curious, he opened her up. To his amazement, the monkey's liver and intestines were bleeding profusely. Apparently, the stress and horror of seeing her child slaughtered had caused her to rupture and bleed from her organs.

"You are deeply distressed and depressed," I told Thomas. "What happened to that mother monkey could happen to you. You have much emotional unbalance in your body at this time, and your sickness is caused by emotional unbalance. Tell me, what has made you so sick?"

Thomas told me his story.

"I have lost almost everything," he said. "My father found out he had cancer and passed away shortly thereafter. I came home early one day and found my wife in bed with another man. We had been married seventeen years and I never had any suspicion that there were any problems. Now she has left me.

"About a month ago my son was killed in an automobile accident. He was only seventeen. Before he died, we found out that our twelve-year-old daughter has leukemia. Now my mother has collapsed and is in the hospital for heart problems.

"On top of that, my accountant stole money from the clinic instead of paying taxes to the Internal Revenue Service. Now the IRS wants to come in and shut the clinic down."

I felt sorry for Thomas. When bad things start happening they are sometimes hard to stop. However, I knew that he could recover from his losses. He was a good doctor and could overcome many of these setbacks if only he could get the stress out of his life.

I administered external Qi Gong to help him achieve the

emotional release that would get rid of the pent-up anger held in his liver. He cried for the next two hours in the treatment room, which was something he definitely needed.

I explained to him that the Chinese believe there are seven human emotions that are related to our internal organs in different ways. The emotion joy effects the heart, while anger affects the liver. Worry gathers in the lungs, stressful thinking in the spleen, sadness in the heart meridian, fear in the kidneys, and shock in the gallbladder. These are normal responses of the body and do not usually cause disease. However, severe or continuous or abruptly occurring emotional stimuli can adversely affect the human body. When this happens, an emotional imbalance takes place. That is when Qi Gong exercises and other forms of treatment should be administered to harmonize the imbalance.

Since Thomas's stress and depression was so great, I decided to treat him for a long period of time, giving him exercises and prescriptions that would balance all seven of his emotions.

Exercises for Harmony

As always, the Golden Eight Exercises are excellent balancing exercises to create internal harmony. But there are a number of extra exercises aimed at taking your mind off of your problems and at cultivating the vital energy that you need to overcome stress and depression. I have included two here. These are simple yet effective means of getting rid of the bad Qi and replenishing the good.

Depression Fighter (Figure 15-1)

Standing straight with your feet shoulder-width apart, close your eyes and press the tip of your tongue against the roof of your mouth. Concentrate on your *dan tien*, the area between your belly button and pubic region. Use only abdominal respiration, in which you breath with your stomach, not your chest.

Without moving your right foot, pivot on your left foot so your left foot is perpendicular to the right, making a T shape (a). Turn toward your left foot.

Inhale and stretch your left arm forward with your palm facing upward, and turn your body to the left as much as possible (b). Then return to the starting position, with your feet parallel. Repeat seven times with the left foot pivoting and then seven times with the right foot pivoting and extending your right arm.

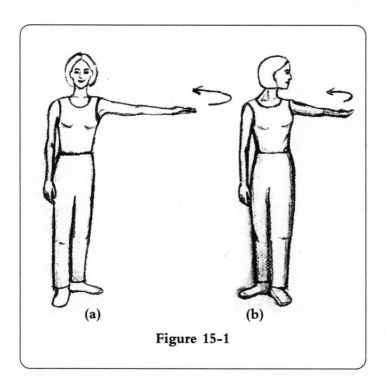

(a)   **(b)**

Figure 15-1

PURPOSE AND EFFECT: This exercise stimulates the meridian channels, striking them almost as you would if you were strumming the strings of a guitar to tune them. Using the same analogy, the *dan tien* is like the guitar body, in that it receives the energy of the Qi channels and vibrates it out to the rest of the body. That is why it is important to breathe with your abdomen during this exercise.

Egyptian King Stress Relief (Figure 15-2)

Sit on the edge of a hard chair with your feet flat on the floor and your hands resting on your kneecaps. Close your eyes and press your tongue against the roof of your mouth and breathe with your abdomen. Focus on your Yong Quan point, located in the arch of the man's left foot and the woman's right foot. Sit in this position for five to ten minutes, remembering to smile as you focus on that spot.

We call this the Egyptian King because a person practicing it looks regal and calm like the stone statues of pharaohs found in the temples of the Nile.

PURPOSE AND EFFECT: When the mind is focused on the foot, it can rest and let the stress drain away. When you have a smile, good energy is distributed to all parts of the body.

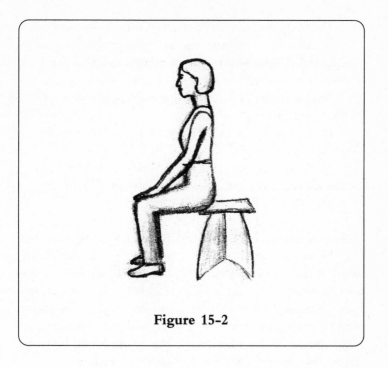

Figure 15-2

HERBS TO BALANCE THE
SEVEN EMOTIONS

The Chinese believe that we have seven emotions. When these emotions are expressed appropriately, they are considered to be in balance. It is when they somehow become out of balance that we have problems. For instance, too much anger can cause energy to rise, while self-doubt can cause energy levels to drop. Joy can cause energy to be lost while sorrow can cause it to stop altogether. Fear can cause energy to freeze or just sink into the lower portions of your body.

The ancient physician Wang Ping explained the interaction of emotions this way:

Joy is the emotion of the heart, which then influences the lungs, leaving the heart unprotected; thus influences of the kidneys are permitted to come to the fore.

Fear is the emotion of the kidneys, and influences the heart, leaving the kidneys unprotected; thus the influences of the spleen are permitted to come to the fore.

Sorrow is the emotion of the liver, and influences the spleen, leaving the liver unprotected; thus influences of the heart come to the fore.

As you can see, the interaction between the mind and the body plays a significant role in the Chinese concept of disease. For many years we were ridiculed by Western medicine for our belief that emotions can manifest themselves as disease. Now, of course, that has changed, with many major medical institutions examining the connection between the mind and body. This illustrates another connection between traditional Chinese beliefs and modern medicine.

The herbal remedy that follows represents the standard treatment for balancing the seven emotions.

Dragon's Bone Decoction

15 grams	Dragon's bone (Long Gu)
15 grams	Oyster shell (Mu Li)
15 grams	Rehmannia root (Di Huang)
15 grams	Ginseng (Ren Shen)
6 grams	Poria (Fu Ling)
6 grams	Biota seed (Bai Zi Ren)
6 grams	Ziziphus (Zsao Ren)
3 grams	Schisandra fruit (Wu Wei Zi)
3 grams	Chaenomeles, dried (Mu Gua)

Preparation and prescription: Combine the herbs in a pot and cover them with filtered water. Then boil the mixture for five minutes. Strain one cup of liquid from this decoction and set aside for later.

Add three more cups of water to the original mixture and boil it until there is about one cup of thick tea. Strain this thick tea from the herbs and combine it in a container with the cup of tea separated earlier.

Drink one cup of the decoction in the morning and another in the afternoon, around four o'clock. Since these herbs can be hard on the stomach lining, it is best to eat something with the tea.

How it works: This oddly named decoction combines ingredients that greatly affect the seven emotions, balancing them to stave off depression and the stress that can cause it.

Dragon's bone in combination with oyster shell and ziziphus are sedative, and are sometimes prescribed alone as a sleeping aid. Rehmannia root and ginseng are added to improve the function of the kidneys and the spleen, which help eliminate some of the toxins in the blood that build up as a result of stress. A large body of research on ginseng tends to back up the Chinese belief that this herb stimulates the central nervous system. A variety of experiments carried out in the Soviet Union since 1948 on athletes and factory workers have shown that ginseng improves endurance and concentration. The Soviet findings were confirmed by the British, who found that hospital nurses reported having greater endurance and concentration when given daily doses of ginseng.

The stimulating effects of ginseng (Ren Shen) are in keeping with its myth, a story of survival in a frozen wilderness. In ancient China, two brothers went deep into the mountains to hunt wild game. It was winter, and they were warned by their parents that a severe storm might trap them in the wilds.

They were young, however, and gave no heed to the warning. When a storm hit, they were far into the mountains and could not return home. All they could do was take shelter in a cave and wait for better weather. After several days, they ran out of food and became extremely hungry. Out of desperation, they began to eat some oddly shaped roots that looked as though they had arms and legs.

"These look like humans," declared one of the brothers.

"Then we must eat our fellow man," said the other brother.

They named the root Ren Shen, which means human form. For several weeks they ate nothing but the roots.

When the snow cleared they returned home, looking robust and healthy. When asked how they survived, one of the brothers pulled a piece of Ren Shen from his bag.

"We ate these little people," he said.

To this day, ginseng is thought to contain human spirits that awaken at night. Because of that, herb collectors tie ginseng with red thread to keep it from running away.

As a contrast, the biota seed and the schisandra fruit act to slow the heart rate and steady the pulse. Schisandra, by the way, has been studied by the Japanese for the protective effect it has on the liver. In their research, they found chemicals called lignins that were extremely effective in protecting the liver from certain toxins. Advocates of this herb have said that it acts as a body tonic to produce energy, but there is no real research to prove this, only hundreds of years of successful use.

The dried chaenomeles (quince) acts to force bad energy down, away from the brain, where it might be causing too much negative activity.

EATING THE BLUES AWAY

Stress leaves the body vulnerable to many things, including illness and poor digestion. Eating is important in staving off the effects and causes of stress and depression. In addition, eating is just plain fun. The following is one of the most effective and enjoyable recipes I know for fighting the blues.

Scampi with Fine Chinese Herbs

¼ ounce	Codonopsis (Dang Shen)
¼ ounce	Angelica (Dang Gui)
15 grams	Lycium fruit (Gou Qi Zi)
15 pieces	Red dates
¼ cup	Rice wine
20 pieces	Shrimp, raw and shelled
1 clove	Garlic, minced
1 tablespoon	Shallots, finely chopped
½ tablespoon	Ginger, finely chopped
½ teaspoon	White pepper
1 teaspoon	Honey
1 tablespoon	Lemon juice
1 teaspoon	Salt
1 tablespoon	Cornstarch
3 tablespoons	Sesame oil

Preparation and prescription: Combine the herbs in rice wine overnight. Strain out the juice and set it aside.

Butterfly the shrimp and combine them in a bowl with the lemon juice, salt, honey, pepper, and cornstarch.

Heat the sesame oil in a skillet and sauté the garlic, shallots, and ginger until they are brown. Then add the shrimp, lycium fruit, and red dates and sauté for two minutes.

Add the herb juice to the shrimp and bring the mixture to high heat for three minutes or until the shrimp is done.

How it works: Stress and depression lead to poor nervous function and reduced blood flow, which must be reversed in order for this condition to go away. This scampi dish is combined with herbs that help improve blood circulation and stimulate the central nervous system. Codonopsis is used in Chinese medicine as a means of replenishing the vital energy of the spleen and lungs, while angelica is combined with wine to invigorate blood circulation. The lycium fruit is added as an anti-aging ingredient because of its antioxidant properties, and red dates, besides being a tasty addition, are considered "protectors of the liver" in traditional Chinese medicine.

In the great tradition of yin and yang, Thomas's life has taken a turn for the better. The exercise and herbs I prescribed helped him get back into balance. His daughter is in full remission from her cancer, thanks to a treatment program that combined both Eastern and Western medicine. He has regained his vigor and has a new girlfriend. The IRS has put him on a monthly payment program to let him pay his back taxes, and he has opened another clinic, one that is smaller and less complicated to manage.

Like all diseases, stress and depression are manifestations of a life out of balance, which the Yellow Emperor had much to say about in his *Classic of Internal Medicine*. At one time, he said, the world was inhabited by "Sages," who did not take things of the world so seriously. As he described them:

> They were able to adjust their desires to worldly affairs, and within their hearts there was neither hatred nor anger. . . . They did not over-exert their bodies at physical labor and they did not over-exert their minds

by strenuous meditation. They were not concerned about anything, they regarded inner happiness and peace as fundamental, and contentment as highest achievement. Their bodies could never be harmed and their mental faculties never be dissipated. Thus they could reach the age of one hundred years or more.

That is some of the best advice I know for overcoming stress and depression.

16

Stroke

A number of medical studies have shown Qi Gong to be an extremely effective method of preventing strokes. One such study was even able to compare its effectiveness to that of a typical Western treatment. In that study, 242 patients with high blood pressure (a common cause of stroke) were divided into two groups. Both groups were given a small dosage of anti-hypertensive drugs. Only one group was treated with Qi Gong. The physicians doing the study then kept track of these patients for thirty years.

By the end of the study, the death rate in the group receiving regular Western treatment was twice that of the Qi Gong group. The group receiving only Western treatment was twice as likely to have high blood pressure as the group receiving Qi Gong and Western treatment.

That Qi Gong can prevent stroke is no surprise to me. Neither is the evidence that it can reverse the effects of a stroke. After all, Qi Gong restores both blood and energy flow, the two vital factors that have been disrupted by a stroke.

There are essentially two types of strokes. In the hemor-rhage variety, an artery has ruptured in the brain, letting the blood spill out into the surrounding tissue. The other type of stroke involves some kind of narrowing of an artery (called thrombosis) or a full blockage of blood (called embolism). This variety takes place when the arteries become narrow from atherosclerosis or when a blood clot breaks loose from another part of the body and travels to the brain.

Western treatment typically prescribes antihypertensive drugs to reduce blood pressure, and anticoagulant drugs to reduce the risk of a stroke caused by a blood clot.

Treatment in China is somewhat different. We combine internal and external Qi Gong with herbal medicines to fight this frightening disease on all fronts. Research has shown that patients who practice Qi Gong exercises respond better to hypertensive drugs, have more efficient heart func-tion, and have blood that is less "sticky" and less likely to clot and cause a blockage.

Let me tell you about one of my case studies.

One day I received a frantic telephone call from one of my apprentices, a man I'll call Tom. He was weeping as he told me about his mother, Nancy. He had found her unconscious on the floor of her home and rushed her to the hospital. Tests revealed that she had fallen victim to a stroke and that her sit-uation was extremely severe. A large portion of her brain was not functional due to the stroke. A type of surgery was sug-gested to stop the bleeding in her brain, but the doctors gave her only a ten percent chance of pulling through the opera-tion alive. Whether surgery was performed or not, the doctors gave her no chance of living as anything but a vegetable.

With little hope offered from Western doctors, Tom decided that his mother should not have the surgery. Instead, he called me. From that day on, I administered external Qi Gong treatments daily.

Within two weeks, Nancy awoke from her coma but was only able to move her fingers. I continued to administer external Qi Gong treatments and added massage, especially of her hands and arms, to help stimulate the nerves that were obviously working. Massage is a simple but powerful tool in fighting many diseases. This is especially true of hand massage. The theory in Chinese medicine it that all of the organs have meridian channels that are connected to the hands and fingers. Therefore, hand massage is like massaging the organs of the entire body.

A good way to massage the hand is to hold the patient's open hand in yours and then run the thumb of your free hand down the entire length of each finger. Do this by pressing your thumb into the base of the palm and then pushing it all the way to the top of each finger. When you reach the end, bend the finger back slightly to allow for a full stretch. Repeat this with each finger of each hand. It is tremendously relaxing and stimulating at the same time.

I also had her perform some of the exercises listed below, especially those that helped her direct her internal Qi, as she gradually regained mobility during her hospital stay.

Exercises like these are important. Not only do they help direct a patient's Qi to an area that needs healing, they also give the patient a sense of control over her disease. This is especially important in stroke victims, who are often left feeling helpless because of their disease. In Chinese medicine, the patient is taught that the cure for an illness will not be accomplished entirely by medicine. The patient can have a great effect upon her illness, too. No matter how grave the situation, I always include the patient in her own treatment.

Tom's mother continued to improve. A month later, she left the hospital. Now she can talk, eat by herself, and even walk with the help of a walker.

She is a good patient and regularly performs Qi Gong exercises. She also takes the daily herbal tea remedy that I prescribed for her. Because of this, she is recovering from a stroke that was supposed to have completely impaired her.

EXERCISE FOR DIRECTING ENERGY

Loss of muscle control is perhaps the most common effect of a stroke. In China, Qi Gong is a common form of therapy for regaining the use of the body. Here is a commonly prescribed set of Qi Gong face and head exercises.

Facial Strength Exercises (Figure 16-1)

Hold your eyes open wide and rotate them clockwise and then counterclockwise, thirty-six times each way. Since the eyes are the gateway to the liver, this will stimulate that organ.

Place the palms of your hands over your ears and spread your fingers horizontally across the back of your head. Now take the index finger of your right hand and place it over the middle finger of your left hand. Push hard on the middle finger until the index finger slides off and "snaps" down on the base of your skull. Repeat this thirty-six times. Since all of the nerves of the body join the brain at that point, this stimulates the entire nervous system.

Smile widely, showing all of your teeth. Tense the neck area at the same time by raising your left shoulder to your ear for a few seconds and then your right shoulder. Now bounce your teeth lightly together thirty-six times. This exercise affects the kidney meridian by improving the flow of good Qi to the kidneys.

Consciously swallow three times to stimulate the production of saliva. Saliva contains important immunoglobin enzymes that combat disease in your body.

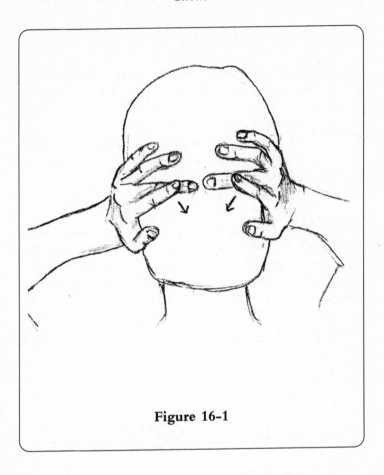

Figure 16-1

PURPOSE AND EFFECT: Since most strokes involve the loss of the body's large movements, Chinese medicine focuses on the small movements, primarily of the face. This is done because all meridian channels travel through the face and head. By performing face and head exercises, you can stimulate all of the meridians and affect all of the internal organs.

Meridian Massage (Figure 16-2)

Since the fingertips are the beginning of the meridians, finger exercises like these can stimulate and even open blocked meridians.

Hold your hand straight out with your palms facing the ground. Raise one digit at a time, beginning with the thumb, up to the upper limit and then down to the lower limit (a, b). Each finger should take about one minute.

Perform this movement with each finger of each hand.

PURPOSE AND EFFECT: Strokes often result in a loss of muscle control. By performing these exercises and putting the fingers through a range of motion one at a time, you will gain a greater level of hand control. These movements also correspond to meridian points that are connected to the internal organs. Stimulating these points can help clear the meridian blockage caused by strokes, providing improved muscle control.

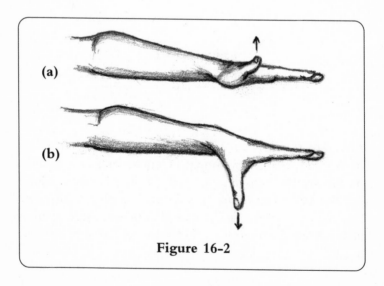

(a)

(b)

Figure 16-2

HERBS FOR STROKE PREVENTION AND RECOVERY

In Chinese medicine, there are many herbal formulas for the prevention of and recovery from strokes. This one is formulated specifically for the prevention of strokes, but I have found it effective in recovery as well.

Astragalus Circulation Enhancer

120 grams	Astragalus root (Huang Qi)
6 grams	Cynomorium (Suo Yang)
6 grams	Angelica root (Dang Gui)
6 grams	Pink peony
3 grams	Cnidium (Chaun Xiang)
3 grams	Achyranthes root (Niu Xi)
3 grams	Persica seed (Tao Ren)
3 grams	Carthamus (Hong Hua)
3 grams	Gastrodia tuber (Tian Ma)
3 grams	Chaenomeles fruit (Mu Gua)
3 grams	Earthworms (Di Long)

Preparation and prescription: Combine the herbs and add five cups of water. Boil this mixture for ten minutes and then strain off one cup of liquid. Save this cup for later.

To the original mixture of herbs, add another three cups of water and boil until there is only about one cup of liquid remaining. Strain the herbs from this thick tea and add the first cup of tea. Separate this mixture into two cups.

For stroke prevention, you should take one dose of this formula per month. Take the first cup at approximately nine in the morning and the second cup at four in the afternoon. Do not drink these on an empty stomach. To recover from a stroke, take one dose every three days.

CAUTION: This is for strokes caused by blockages like blood clots. Do not take this medication if your stroke is caused by a hemorrhage, like a broken blood vessel.

How it works: This decoction dissolves clots and improves circulation while stimulating the central nervous system, which provides overall energy. The main clot-buster in this formula is the achyranthes. Frequently used as an herbal method of clearing bruises of pooled blood, this plant has long been used as a means of dissolving clots and improving circulation. This herb and pink peony combine to stimulate liver function and improve circulation.

In Chinese medicine, astragalus is almost always combined with angelica when poor circulation is involved. The main effect of astragalus is to enhance the immune system, but angelica has the greatest effect upon blood circulation. Angelica is widely known as the tonic for female disorders. Because it contains estrogen compounds, it is an effective way of regulating menstrual periods and dealing with premenstrual syndrome. It is also given as a cure for vaginal yeast infections and as a means of controlling some fungal infections.

Angelica's anti-cancer properties fall into the realm of immunity enhancers. Medical tests in China and Japan have shown that this herb stimulates the production of white blood cells as well as the production of interferon. In animal studies, it has been shown to inhibit the formation of skin tumors. Angelica is readily available in a capsule formula called Dang Gui. It is more effective, however, if taken in decoction form.

Angelica is effective in use with strokes because of its vasodilator effects, probably due to a class of chemicals it contains called coumarins. Not only do these chemicals relax arteries, they are also used as antispasmodics, which means they can keep arteries from cramping and causing what is known as transient ischemic attacks, or "little" strokes. The chemicals in angelica (Dang Gui) also make it a stimulant to the central nervous system, which is part of the beautiful myth about the origin of this herb.

According to this myth, a young man was bow hunting when he noticed a beautiful falcon resting on a huge chestnut tree. As he took aim at the bird, it began to speak to him in human language, begging him not to fire the arrow.

"My mother is blind and needs me to provide food," said the falcon. "If you let me go, I will provide you with some seeds of a medicinal herb."

The young man was touched and he lowered his bow. As promised, the bird spat a drop of blood containing seeds of a medicinal herb and then flew away.

The man planted the seeds, and three days later, a plant began to grow with sturdy stems and blood-red flowers. When the young man ate the plant, he felt invigorated and robust. He gave portions of the plant to other villagers. Those who were sick became well, and those who were not sick felt energized, as the young man had.

All the while, small birds flew around his hut screeching, "Dang gui, dang gui!" From that day forward, the plant was referred to by the name the tiny screeching birds had given it.

STROKE-FIGHTING FOODS

Since it is poor diet that leads to many cases of hypertension and strokes, it makes sense that good diet can improve the conditions that lead to these problems.

Doctors in the West are encouraged by organizations like the American Heart Association to make dietary change a form of treatment for vascular diseases. In China, where food is an effective form of medicine, we have already done this for more than three thousand years.

There are many recipes for the treatment of strokes and hypertension in the Chinese kitchen, so I will not attempt to cover them all. Here are two recipes that are aimed at the treatment and prevention of strokes.

Beef with Herbs

10 grams	Polygonatum Cirrhifolium (Huang Jing)
10 grams	Astragalus (Huang Qi)
½ teaspoon	Ginger (sliced)
3 cups	Water
½ pound	Lean beef (sliced)
3 pieces	Scallions

Preparation and prescription: Simmer the Huang Jing, astragalus, and ginger in the water for thirty minutes in a covered pan. Pour through a strainer and save the juice.

In a separate pan, combine the juice with the beef and the scallions. Simmer over a slow heat for thirty minutes. Add salt and pepper to taste and a dash of cooking wine.

How it works: This dish is good for restoring general strength to the body. Astragalus also has properties that improve blood circulation in a number of areas of the body, including the brain. In addition to adding a sweet flavor to this dish, polygonatum has the reputation in China of being an herb for longevity. In some of the lore of the Orient, it is written that eating the root of this plant allowed an old man to father five children. In one of China's early medical texts, it is written that "If one uses Golden Essence [polygonatum] for only one year, the old will become young again."

Corn Silk Bean Curd Soup

4 ounces	Corn silk (available at Chinese markets)
5 cups	Water
½ pound	Bean curd (diced)
1 cup	Shiitake mushrooms (sliced)
1 tablespoon	Sesame oil
1	Scallion (chopped)
1 tablespoon	Cornstarch

Preparation and prescription: Boil corn silk for fifteen minutes. Strain and save the juice.

Put the juice in a pot and add all the ingredients *except* the cornstarch. Mix the cornstarch in cold water and stir into the soup. Add salt and pepper to taste, heat and serve.

How it works: Corn silk's main medicinal strength is its ability to cleanse the blood of cholesterol. Add to that its cleansing effects on the liver and you have a food that can both rejuvenate and strengthen the vascular system.

Strokes require more perseverance than most other diseases, mainly because of the loss of motor and mental skills. This can lead to a great amount of frustration on the part of both patient and caretaker. When I deal with stroke victims and their families, I remind them of the need to be patient and uplifting, and frequently read them these words from the Yellow Emperor about the need for spirit: "Nowadays vitality and energy are considered the foundation of life. . . . How can a disease be cured when there is no spiritual energy within the body?"

17

Weight Loss

The emperors of ancient China were given to many excesses, including rich food and too much leisure time. Those in the royal court were the only ones in society who had such excesses, so fat and softness became a sign of wealth all over China. Even though fat was a sign of wealth, it was certainly not a sign of health. Chinese physicians have always warned of the dangers of the "high fat" lifestyle. In 1330, a physician named Hu Sihui published *Important Principles of Food and Drink*, which championed the idea that good health comes from a balanced diet. "[The ancient people] took as their guide to life the harmony between yin and yang," he wrote. "[Today's people] are ignorant of what to avoid in their diet, and they pay no heed to moderation."

Even earlier than that, a royal lifestyle was blamed for illness. In the first century, the emperor asked Guo Yu, the royal physician, why he was more effective in healing "ordinary people" than the privileged. The physician's answer was surprisingly blunt. "Because the privileged have a love of idleness and a dislike of work," he said. "And they do not take care of their bodies."

I told these stories to one of my weight-loss patients, who had a "royal body," and she shrugged. "I don't lead a royal lifestyle," she said. "I work eight hours a day and I don't have time for much else. Between family, work, and commuting, I don't have time to look after my body."

"That is correct," I said to the woman. "But the effect is the same. You become physically inactive just like ancient royalty. The rigors of everyday living lead you to eat for comfort and stress relief. Although the lifestyle is different, you still become overweight, overstressed, and underexercised. Soon, you develop a royal body."

Modern science has proven that being overweight leads to a number of health concerns, including heart disease, stroke, hypertension, diabetes, gout, and even cancer. All of the world's medical systems consider extra weight a major health risk. In Chinese medicine, a person who is ten percent heavier than normal is overweight, while a person who is twenty percent heavier is considered extremely unhealthy.

WEIGHT LOSS EXERCISES

The mind is a key factor in weight loss. I tell my weight-loss patients that a leaner body is the product of a calm mind. I also understand that calmness is not always easy in our fast-paced world. To remain successful, we are required to work fast, which leads to anxieties that we too often try to quell with food.

The exercises that follow help break that cycle of weight gain. Not only are they meditative, but they also have a direct physiological effect on the factors that make you hungry. The following exercises are not active ones like the Golden Eight. They are meditative in nature, aimed at calming your anxiety while staving off hunger.

I recommend doing these exercises in conjunction with the Golden Eight Exercises. In fact, since exercise is such an important component of weight loss, I have my weight-loss patients practice the Golden Eight twice a day.

Turbulent Wave (Figure 17-1)

Practice this exercise only when you feel hungry. Because the movement resembles an ocean wave, this is called Turbulent Wave. This exercise can be done standing.

Standing straight with your knees slightly bent, put one hand on your chest and the other on your lower abdomen (a).

As you breathe in, expand your chest and contract your stomach (b). As you breathe out, raise your abdomen as high as possible and contract your chest (c).

Repeat this forty times. One repetition consists of one inhalation and one exhalation. In most cases the feeling of hunger will disappear. If you still feel hungry, do another twenty repetitions. This should solve the problem in most cases.

Since doing this too fast may cause dizziness, it is important to do this exercise at a rate of breathing that is close to your normal rate of respiration.

PURPOSE AND EFFECT: Very few people still feel hunger after doing this exercise. The reason for the loss of hunger is the change this exercise brings about in your stomach's acidity. Hunger pains are caused by digestive juices stimulating the mucus membranes of the stomach wall. When you do the Turbulent Wave, stomach acid is forced down and out of your stomach, which greatly reduces the feelings of hunger. With the belly breathing involved, the stomach expands and is less inclined to produce acids.

Although this exercise is usually done as a means to keep from eating, it can also be used to keep from eating *too much*. To dull your appetite, practice the Turbulent Wave before each meal.

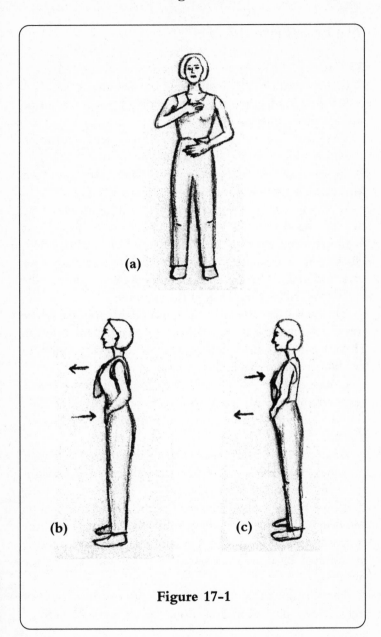

Figure 17-1

The Frog (Figure 17-2)

This is a good exercise to practice when your hunger is caused by stress or by a sudden drop in blood sugar. It is called the Frog because the person doing it resembles a frog sitting quietly on a riverbank.

To do this exercise, sit on a chair or sofa, with your thigh and lower leg forming an angle of ninety degrees or less. Remove glasses and all jewelry and loosen your belt. Your knees should be about shoulder-width apart.

If you are a woman, make a fist of your left hand and wrap the right hand around it. If you are a man, make a fist of your right hand and wrap your left hand around it (a). Place both elbows on your knees and lower your forehead onto your clenched hands. Close your eyes and relax your entire body.

Exhale, as if sighing from great fatigue.

Then visualize the most beautiful sight possible. Make sure it is something that makes you feel happy and peaceful. Hold this image for a minute or two, to coax your mind into reaching a state of happiness and contentment.

Once you have reached this deeply relaxed state, concentrate entirely on the action of your breathing. Not even thunder should disturb you as you breathe slowly and comfortably.

After a few relaxing breaths, begin to breathe with your abdomen. Take half a breath into your abdomen and hold it for a few seconds before exhaling (b, c). Repeat this belly breathing for about five minutes, making sure not to breathe too deeply or to use your chest. Some people are made dizzy by this breathing technique. After doing it a couple of times, you should become accustomed to it and not experience dizziness.

Then imagine that your body's energy, or Qi, is a ball of light. Move this ball of light from the top or your head to

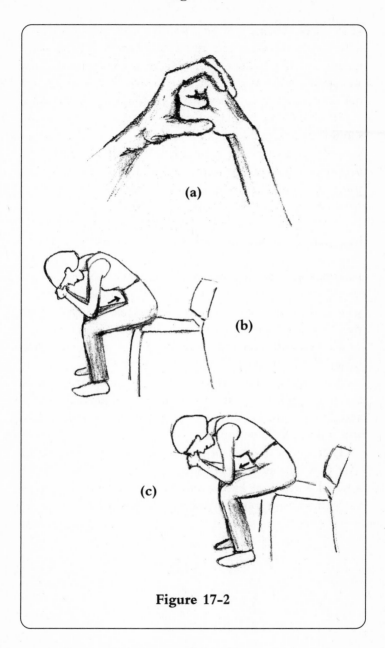

Figure 17-2

your lower abdomen, or *dan tien*. Then imagine this ball of light moving up from your feet to your *dan tien*. Then imagine the ball of light moving up your arms, through your body and into your *dan tien*. Finally, imagine this light energy coming through all of your pores and going into your *dan tien*.

The breathing and visualization portion of this exercise should take ten to fifteen minutes. When you are finished, lift your head slowly with your eyes closed. Rub your hands together to make them warm, and "wash" your face with the palms of your hands to provide an enlivening massage. Then open your eyes and stretch like a cat.

Practice this three times a day before meals. You will be in high spirits, and your appetite will be lessened.

PURPOSE AND EFFECT: When you practice the Frog, blood and Qi are forced into your head, limbs, and other parts of your body, which reduces their need for blood sugar, which may have been the source of your hunger to begin with.

This exercise also has a calming effect upon the mind, which also may have been the source of the hunger to begin with. I call this "false hunger" because it is generally caused by anxiety, not a true need for food. Through visualization and deep breathing, this anxiety can usually be eliminated and, with it, the false hunger.

There are a number of positive side effects of the Frog. The position and deep breathing provide massage of the internal organs. The exercise also improves your lung capacity by increasing your diaphragm's range of motion.

HERBAL REMEDIES FOR WEIGHT LOSS

There are many different reasons for weight gain, but the bottom line is that most people simply eat too much. The following are herbal formulas that reduce a person's hunger through different actions. This first formula reduces hunger while altering the metabolism to make a person a more efficient fat burner.

Ten-Herb Decoction for Weight Loss

15 grams	Rhaponticum root (Lou Lu)
15 grams	Cassia seed (Jue Ming Zi)
15 grams	Alisma tuber (Ze Xie)
15 grams	Lotus leaf (Hugh Ye)
15 grams	Stephania root (Fang Ji)
15 grams	Rehmannia root (Sheng Di)
6 grams	Red ginseng (Hong Sen)
30 grams	Black beans
30 grams	Ephedra root (Ling Yang Gen)
30 grams	Coix seed (Yi Mi)

Preparation and prescription: Combine all the herbs in a pot and cover with filtered water. Boil the mixture for five minutes. Then strain off one cup of liquid and set it aside for later use.

To the original mixture of herbs, add another three cups of water and boil this mixture until there is only about one cup of liquid remaining in the pot. Strain the liquid from the thick herbs and mix this second cup with the liquid from the first cup. You will now have two cups of Ten-Herb Decoction tea.

Drink one cup in the morning at about nine and the other in the afternoon about four. Be sure to eat before drinking this herbal tea.

I recommend this formula for up to ten weeks.

How it works: The Chinese have tested this formula in clinical trials with obese patients and have found that, in conjunction with moderation in diet, it leads to an average weight loss of twenty-five pounds in ten weeks. The combination of herbs in this formula is aimed at making the metabolism more efficient. It does this in a number of ways. For example, the combination of alisma tuber, rehmannia root, stephania root, black bean, and coix seed helps rid the body of dampness and excess water. Separately, they act on different organs. The coix seed makes the spleen function more effectively, while the black bean provides nourishment to the kidneys. The stephenia root acts as a diuretic to rid the body of excess water, which is necessary because the spleen and kidneys are too yin, or passive.

In Chinese medicine, being overweight can sometimes be caused by organs that are too active, or have too much heat. To eliminate heat in the liver, I combined cassia seed, rhaponticum root, and ephedra root. Each of these works in its own way to eliminate fire from the liver. Cassia seed, for instance, lowers both blood pressure and blood cholesterol, while the ephedra root clears toxins from the bloodstream. Lotus leaf is added to dispel heat in the liver and spleen. Finally, red ginseng is added as an energy booster. This is done because most people who are overweight complain of not having enough energy. This provides them with more Qi.

Diet Tea

36 grams	Coix seed (Yi Mi)
36 grams	Pinellia (Ban Xia)
36 grams	Tangerine peel (Chen Pi)
36 grams	Areca peel (Da Fu Pi)

Preparation and prescription: Combine the herbs in a pot and cover with filtered water. Boil the mixture for five minutes, then strain off one cup of liquid and set it aside for later use.

To the original mixture of herbs, add another three cups of water and boil this mixture until there is only about one cup of liquid remaining in the pot.

Strain the liquid from the thick herbs and mix this second cup with the liquid from the first cup. You will now have two cups of the diet tea.

Drink one cup in the morning at about nine and the other in the afternoon at about four. Be sure to eat before drinking this tea to avoid stomach upset.

How it works: In China this diet tea was tested on more than one hundred obese patients. Within ten weeks, seventy-five percent of them had experienced serious weight loss, which was defined as losing more than twenty pounds.

The weight loss was caused by the appetite-reducing effects of the herbs. This formula works on the metabolism by eliminating excess dampness and promoting the flow of Qi energy to various organs. The combination of coix seed, tangerine peel, and areca peel has a diuretic effect as well as an energizing effect on the stomach and spleen. The pinellia and the tangerine remove mucus from the body as well. When excess water and mucus are removed, the metabolism burns calories more effectively.

This formula also reduces hunger.

HEALTHY DISHES FOR WEIGHT LOSS

"Take care with [your] words," says the *Book of Changes*. "And be moderate in eating and drinking."

Unfortunately, people who are eating in moderation

because they are trying to lose weight usually do not have kind words to say about their food. Most diet food is bland and virtually tasteless, which amounts to a loss of pleasure.

I understand that it is important to keep some of the pleasure of eating, which is why I have included two of my favorite healthy dishes. Both of these are low in fat and cholesterol while being high in vitamins and taste.

Bamboo Ginseng Chicken Soup

1½ cups	Chicken broth
1 cup	Water
½ cup	Bamboo ginseng (Zhu Shen)
5 stalks	Asparagus
1 tablespoon	Sesame oil
2 pieces	Green onion, cut into one-inch lengths
1 clove	Garlic, sliced
1 teaspoon	Ginger, sliced

Preparation and prescription: Soak the bamboo ginseng in boiling water for ten minutes.

Blanch the asparagus in boiling water for one minute. Drain and set aside.

Heat the sesame oil in a pot and sauté the garlic and ginger until they are aromatic. Then add the chicken broth and water and heat until they simmer.

Add the bamboo ginseng and let it cook for five minutes. Then add the asparagus and let it cook for another minute. Finally, add the green onions and serve.

How it works: As a meal, this simple soup is tasty, satisfying, and low-fat. This recipe makes two servings with only ninety-nine calories each. Yet it is high in protein as well as vitamins B, C, and E.

Shiitake Mushrooms in Oyster Sauce

8 ounces	Fresh shiitake mushrooms (without stalks)
1	Carrot, sliced, cooked for one minute
1 head	Lettuce
1 teaspoon	Salt
½ teaspoon	Honey
3 teaspoons	Corn oil, divided
1	Shallot, sliced
2 cloves	Garlic, sliced
2 tablespoons	Oyster sauce
1 teaspoon	Wine

Preparation and prescription: Combine the mushrooms with the salt, honey, and two teaspoons of corn oil. Cook this combination for fifteen minutes and set aside.

Blanch the lettuce in two cups of boiling water for thirty seconds and drain. Then arrange the lettuce leaves on a platter.

Heat one teaspoon of corn oil and sauté the shallots and garlic until aromatic. Then add the steamed mushrooms with the stock, oyster sauce, wine, and sliced carrots. Cook for two minutes until the mixture thickens.

Spoon the mixture over the lettuce and serve.

How it works: Low in fat yet high in healing properties, this recipe, which serves two, contains only 340 calories per serving. Its most active ingredient is the shiitake mushroom. Research shows that shiitake can boost immunity and fight viruses. But this wonderful mushroom has an added benefit for the person trying to lose weight. Japanese researchers found that eating three ounces of fresh shiitake a day resulted in a twelve percent reduction in serum cholesterol in test subjects. Not only is this dish helping you lose weight, it is also cleaning out your arteries.

I have conducted many weight-loss programs at corporations in the Los Angeles area, and I have had to monitor the participants' progress so the company managers could tell if the programs were worth keeping. With the information I have included here for you, my patients have lost an average of three pounds per week, with many losing even more.

Most important, however, is the new sense of control over their eating reported by many of the participants. Instead of eating from anxiety, they now do the Qi Gong exercises to control their hunger.

Afterword

Each person carries his own doctor inside him. They come to us not knowing that truth. We are at our best when we give the doctor who resides within each patient a chance to go to work.

—ALBERT SCHWEITZER

Even though Qi Gong has been used with great effectiveness for thousands of years, there are still many scientific mysteries about how it works. Gradually, however, those gaps in knowledge are being filled. In China and other parts of the Orient, Qi Gong has been studied by many researchers who have produced thousands of pages of scientific data proving the effectiveness of this healing art. I have referred to many of those studies in this book.

It was not until the 1980s that Qi Gong became the subject of serious research in China. This research was encouraged and funded by the Chinese government to learn why it was so effective. By then, for instance, I had treated more than ten thousand patients and was working in one of China's major hospitals using Qi Gong in conjunction with Western medicine for the treatment of cancer patients. The government was no longer trying to eliminate traditional Chinese medicine; it was trying to understand it. The results of this research have been rich and encouraging, and have led to more questions that can be answered only with further research. The Chinese government now funds a tremendous amount of Qi Gong research. Every few years it even sponsors international conferences for the exchange of such research.

Scientific interest has now spread to the Western medical establishment. Much of the continuing exploration into Qi Gong will be carried out by the National Institutes of Health, most likely by its Office of Alternative Medicine. The NIH has focused on Qi Gong as one form of medicine that it plans to examine more closely by funding research at major medical institutions in the United States.

More specifically, the NIH, in its report *Alternative Medical Systems and Practices in the United States*, cites an interest in studying "emissions from external Qi Gong practitioners" to better understand the nature of the "infrasonic energy" that is present when they practice energetic healing. The NIH has also funded studies of other aspects of Qi Gong that were mentioned in this book, such as the effect of external Qi on cancer cells and the effects of internal Qi on such ailments as hypertension, heart disease, and arthritis.

Many Qi Gong masters laugh at this research. They feel that to spend time and money examining treatments that have proven effective for thousands of years is foolish. I disagree. I am glad to see that the NIH is interested in Qi Gong. It is through such diligent efforts that Qi Gong will be studied and understood by medical doctors in the Western world.

★ ★ ★

Afterword

Despite the current shortage of Western research in Qi Gong, word has spread about its effectiveness. Already many Western physicians have referred patients to me. These referral patients are usually ones who have not responded well to Western medicine and have begun to ask for some kind of alternative solution to their problems. Under these conditions, I jokingly call myself "the doctor for the truly sick," because I am getting patients who have pancreatic cancer, AIDS, multiple sclerosis, brain tumors, heart disease, and other life-threatening problems that Western medicine has failed to help.

These are my favorite patients. They are extremely compliant and are always willing to give the Qi Gong approach one hundred percent of their effort. They all understand that Qi Gong is a discipline that combines isometric exercise, guided imagery, isotonic exercises, meditation, herbs, the body's own chemicals of healing, and a number of other responses that are not yet understood by medicine. They know that, even though the science of Qi Gong is not completely understood, a healing force has been mustered on their behalf that is fighting to bring their body back into proper balance. As users, they have an understanding of Qi Gong that most researchers will never have.

This is why interest in Qi Gong is growing all over the world. People know that not all of the marvels of the human body can be explained by science. There is a driving force that gives us life and health, a force that speaks to that doctor inside each of us. More and more, people are realizing they can master their own miracles by learning healing arts like Qi Gong. They are also understanding what the Taoists meant when they said:

The root of the way of life, of birth and change, is Qi;
the myriad things of heaven and earth all obey this law.
Thus Qi in the periphery envelops heaven and earth.

Qi in the interior activates them. The source wherefrom the sun, moon, and stars derive their light, the thunder, rain, wind and cloud their being, the four seasons and the myriad things their birth, growth, gathering and storing; all this is brought about by Qi. Man's possession of life is completely dependent upon this Qi.

Resources

SUPPLIES AND INFORMATION ABOUT QI GONG

Most of the herbs discussed in this book are available at Chinese pharmacies, which are located in the Chinese districts of almost any moderate- to large-sized city. Other sources of these herbs are Chinese markets and even natural food stores. If you are unable to locate an herb mentioned in this book, or if you would prefer that I prepare the herbal formula for you, fax or write to me at the address below and I will send a price list:

Master Hong Liu
P.O. Box 726
Duarte, CA 91009-0726
FAX: 818-359-7612
E-mail address: miracles@qimaster.com

OTHER SOURCES OF HERBS AND HERBAL REMEDIES

Dragon's Light Herb Company
211 Clayton Street
Denver, CO 80206
303-329-9060

Emperor's College of Traditional Oriental Medicine
1807-B Wilshire Boulevard
Santa Monica, CA 90403
310-453-8300

NOTE: It would be helpful to have the name of the formula and the recipe to refer to when contacting the sources in this list.

VIDEOS

I have two videos available: *Qi Gong for Weight Loss* offers an effective program for weight loss, while *Qi Gong for Healing* offers specific exercises and advice for improving your immunity and vitality. Each video costs $29.95. To order write to:

New Light Productions
P.O. Box 13255
Scottsdale, AZ 85267

or:

Master Hong, Inc.
P.O. Box 726
Duarte, CA 91009-0726
FAX: 818-359-7612

References

There are hundreds of medical studies examining the effects of Qi Gong on various disease states. Included in this list are some of the better studies, many of which were conducted by my colleagues in China. Although this book is based primarily on the results I have achieved in my clinical practice (both in the United States and China), this research represents some of the best science to examine this ancient form of healing.

Achterberg, J., L. Dossey, J. Gordon. February 1, 1993. Report of the panel on mind/body interventions. National Institutes of Health Office of Alternative Medicine.

Bao, G., S. Wei, S. Zhang. 1993. Study of Qigong harmonizing of the human circulation system. Proceedings from the Second World Conference for Academic Exchange of Medical Qigong in Beijing, China.

Bornoroni, C., V. Genitoni, G. Gori, G. Gatti, A. Dorigo. 1993. Treatment of 30 cases of primary hypertension by Qigong techniques. Proceedings from the Second World Conference for Academic Exchange of Medical Qigong in Beijing, China.

Cao, X., T. Ye, Y. Gao. 1988. Anti-tumor metastases activity of emitted Qi in tumor bearing mice. Proceedings from the First World Conference for Academic Exchange of Medical Qigong in Beijing, China.

Feng L. 1988. Effect of emitted Qi on human carcinoma cells. Proceedings from the First World Conference for Academic Exchange of Medical Qigong in Beijing, China.

Feng, L., L. Peng. 1993. Effect of emitted Qi on prevention and treatment of tumors in mice. Proceedings from the Second World Conference for Academic Exchange of Medical Qigong in Beijing, China.

Feng, L., Y. Wang, S. Chen. Effects of emitted Qi on the immune functions of mice. Proceedings from the First World Conference for Academic Exchange of Medical Qigong in Beijing, China.

Feng, L., S. Chen, L. Zhu. 1993. Effect of emitted Qi on the growth of mice. Proceedings from the Second World Conference for Academic Exchange of Medical Qigong in Beijing, China.

Fu, J. 1993. Treatment of advanced gastric cancer in the aged by the combination of Qigong and medicinal herbs. Proceedings from the Second World Conference for Academic Exchange of Medical Qigong in Beijing, China.

Jing, G. 1988. Observations on the curative effects of Qigong self-adjustment therapy in hypertension. Proceedings from the First World Conference for Academic Exchange of Medical Qigong in Beijing, China.

Lei, X. 1992. How external Qi strengthens the anti–tumor immune function. Proceedings from the Third International Qigong Conference in Kyoto, Japan.

Li, Z., L. Li, B. Zhang. 1988. Group observation and experimental research on the prevention and treatment of hypertension by Qigong. Proceedings from the First World Conference for Academic Exchange of Medical Qigong in Beijing, China.

Li, X. 1992. 40 clinical cases of treatment of rheumatoid arthritis by Qigong. Proceedings from the Fourth International Symposium on Qigong in Shanghai, China.

Liu, Y., S. He, S. Xie. 1993. Clinical observation on the treatment of 158 cases of cerebral arteriosclerosis by Qigong. Proceedings from the Second World Conference on Academic Exchange of Medical Qigong in Beijing, China.

Liu, T., M. Wan, O. Lu. 1988. Experiment of emitted Qi on animals. Proceedings from the First World Conference for Academic Exchange of Medical Qigong in Beijing, China.

Liu, D., X. Shen, C. Wang. 1990. Study of the effect of natural killer cell activity to mice with tumor by means of external Qi. Proceedings from the Third International Symposium on Qigong in Shanghai, China.

Liu, Z., J. Wang, J. Ren. 1993. Study of the biological effect of emitted Qi on microbes. Proceedings from the Second World Conference on Academic Exchange of Medical Qigong in Beijing, China.

Machi, Y. 1993. Measurement of physiological phenomena and others of Qigong masters under the Qigong state. Proceedings from the Second World Conference for Academic Exchange of Medical Qigong in Beijing, China.

Mo, F., Y. Xu, Y. Lu, G. Xu. 1993. Study of preventing of cardiac function disorder due to immediate entry into highlands by Qigong exercise. Proceedings from the Second World Conference on Academic Exchange of Medical Qigong in Beijing, China.

Qian, S., W. Sun, Q. Liu, Y. Wan. 1993. Influence of emitted Qi on cancer growth, metastasis and survival time of the host. Proceedings from the Second World Conference for Academic Exchange of Medical Qigong in Beijing, China.

Rubik, R. September 1995. Can Western Science Provide a Foundation for Acupuncture? *Alternative Therapies in Health and Medicine.*

Sancier, K. 1995. Medical applications of Qigong. *Alternative Therapies in Health and Medicine,* 2(1).

Sancier, K., B. Hu. 1991. Medical applications of Qigong and emitted Qi on humans, animals, cell cultures, and plants: Review of selected scientific research. *American Journal of Acupuncture,* 19(4).

Sun, F., Y. Jiao, J. Wang, L. Cheng. 1993. Influence of mental activity on the respiration regulation during Qigong exercise. Proceedings from the Second World Conference for Academic Exchange of Medical Qigong in Beijing, China.

Tang, C., X. Wei. 1993. Effect of Qigong on personality. Proceedings from the Second World Conference for Academic Exchange of Medical Qigong in Beijing, China.

References

Wang, C., D. Xu, Y. Qian. 1990. The beneficial effect of Qigong on the hypertension incorporated with coronary heart disease. Proceedings from the Third international Symposium on Qigong in Shanghai, China.

Wang, C., D. Xu, Y. Qian, W. Shi. 1993. Effects of Qigong on prevention of stroke and alleviating the multiple cerebro-cardiovascular risk factors: a follow up report on 242 hypertensive cases over 30 years. Proceedings from the Second World Conference for Academic Exchange of Medical Qigong in Beijing, China.

Wang, Y. 1993. Clinical observation on 30 cases of cancer treated by Qigong therapy. Proceedings from the Second World Conference for Academic Exchange of Medical Qigong in Beijing, China.

Wu, B., X. Wang, Z. Wang, J. Liu. 1993. The study of magnetic signals under the Qigong state by superconducting bio-magnetometer. Proceedings from the Second World Conference for Academic Exchange of Medical Qigong in Beijing, China.

Xong, J., Z. Lu. 1993. Curative effect on 120 cancer cases treated by Chinese-Western medicine and Qigong therapy. Proceedings from the Second World Conference on Academic Exchange of Medical Qigong in Beijing, China.

Yu, Y., R. Zhang, X. Huang, Y. Guo. 1993. Effect of self-controlling Qigong therapy on the immune function of cancer patients. Proceedings from the Second World Conference on Academic Exchange of Medical Qigong in Beijing, China.

Yuan, Z. 1993. Survey of 100 doctors using simulated Qigong in the USA. Proceedings from the Second World Conference on Academic Exchange of Medical Qigong in Beijing, China.

Zhang, L., L. Wang, Y. Yan. 1993. Adjusting effect of emitted Qi on the immune function of cold-stressed mice. Proceedings from the Second World Conference for Academic Exchange of Medical Qigong in Beijing, China.

Zhao, H., J. Bian. 1993. Curative effect of intelligence Qigong on 122 tumor patients. Proceedings from the Second World Conference for Academic Exchange of Medical Qigong in Beijing, China.

Zhuo, Peiyan. 1989. Preliminary report of treating 32 cases of coronary heart disease by a system of deep breathing exercises. Proceedings from the Second International Conference on Qigong in Xian, China.

About the Author

MASTER HONG LIU became a medical doctor in China with a specialty in the treatment of cancer and an advanced degree in herbal medicine, and he is one of only a small number of Qi Gong masters in the world. He trained for thirty years with renowned Taoist and Shaolin masters, including eight years under the Qi Gong Master Kwan, and treated high-ranking Communist Party members in China. Master Liu served as a distinguished professor of Qi Gong at the Emperor's College of Traditional Oriental Medicine in Santa Monica and Samra University of Oriental Medicine in Los Angeles, and currently maintains professional offices in suburban Los Angeles.

PAUL PERRY is the coauthor of three bestselling books, including *Saved by the Light*. He lives in Scottsdale, Arizona.